Traditional African Bonesetters and Western Medical Practitioners

Traditional African Bonesetters and Western Medical Practitioners

Fractured Patient Care Systems in Cameroon, Ethiopia, Ghana, and Zimbabwe

Roxane E. Richter, Thomas M. Flowers,
Elias K. Bongmba, and Ananya K. Admasu

ANTHEM PRESS

Anthem Press
An imprint of Wimbledon Publishing Company
www.anthempress.com

This edition first published in UK and USA 2026
by ANTHEM PRESS
75–76 Blackfriars Road, London SE1 8HA, UK
or PO Box 9779, London SW19 7ZG, UK
and
244 Madison Ave #116, New York, NY 10016, USA

British Library Cataloguing-in-Publication Data
A catalogue record for this book is available from the British Library.

Library of Congress Cataloging-in-Publication Data: 2026930585

ISBN-13: 978-1-83999-709-9 (Hbk)
ISBN-10: 1-83999-709-5 (Hbk)

Cover credit: Mantas Mozeris

This title is also available as an eBook.

TABLE OF CONTENTS

LIST OF PHOTOS

LIST OF FIGURES AND CHARTS

PREFACE

Traditional Bone Setting (TBS) has long held prominent sway in African healthcare, particularly in the more remote and pastoral expanses of Western, Central, Eastern, and Southern Africa. This unique interdisciplinary religious, human rights, and socio-biological study of medicine manuscript is an examination of not only generationally inherited ethnobotanical/pharmacognosy TBS traditions—but also direct observation(s) on how current surgical orthopedic medicine and modern-day social mechanisms can clash with traditional healthcare approaches in contemporaneous and inexorable ways. Whether intentionally or not, this entrenched two-tier infrastructure supports, promotes, and maintains a fiscally and socially alienated infrastructure: One that serves the underprivileged in the general public; and the other that is oriented toward serving the prosperous, powerful, and upwardly mobile urban class. Some argue these disparate structures are perpetually destined to remain grassroots-based adversaries, due to systemic mistrust, irreconcilable intellectual and spiritual beliefs, and potential biochemical appropriations.

These ensuing biomedical collisions between 'modern Western' orthopedic trauma care and traditional bonesetters in Cameroon (Central Africa), Ethiopia (East Africa), Ghana (West Africa), and Zimbabwe (South Africa) were selected and documented over nine years via several multidisciplinary mechanisms: one-on-one interviews with TBS patients and practicing native bonesetters; in-country practicing orthopedic surgeons; ethnobotanical TBS poultice(s) phytochemical analyses; global health experts; and Western-trained emergency physicians. Other assessments included: fracture treatments (poultice, manipulation, ingested medicines, etc.), evidence-based research on ethnobotanical structures, qualitative patient-recorded preferences of TBS, quantitative complications and casualties inherent in fracture management, modern orthopedic history and challenges in Africa, as well some of the current and future standardizations of alternative medical care practices. Medicinal plants have been utilized (via innumerable structural and functional diversities and extraction techniques) in traditional healthcare systems since prehistoric times—and to this day—remain the singularly most important accessible healthcare resource for the vast majority of the world's population.

Holistic Homeostasis

In Western biomedical quarters, it will continue to be argued that traditional bonesetters' lack of anatomical, physiological, and radiological knowledge effects tragic and unnecessary limb- and/or life-threatening complications. However, in stark contrast to Western medicine—which focuses on the empirical and scientific dissection, analysis, diagnosis, and treatment of singular biological 'organ systems' (respiratory, digestive, circulatory, urinary, integumentary, skeletal, muscular, endocrine, lymphatic, nervous and reproductive) or body parts (ear, nose, or throat) via medical specialties (cardiology, gastroenterology, neurology, etc.)—holistic traditional medicine distinguishes itself to take into consideration the mind-body integrated person in the treatment of injuries and illnesses—physically, psychologically, socially and spiritually. Bishaw[1] in his 1991 studies of indigenous Ethiopian medicine, found that one of traditional medicine's most important contributions may come from its "holistic approach to disease and other human problems," and argued that any attempt to separate the 'empirical' from the 'spiritual' for the purposes of "approaching and incorporating only the 'empirical' into the modern health care system" would inevitably result not in the promotion of traditional medicine, but, on the contrary, in rendering it "as mechanical and segmented as modern medicine may have become of late".[p199] As healthcare providers, we certainly respect the amazing and extraordinary capacities of our human bodies to heal; honestly, sometimes the most important thing we can "do" is to just get out of the way of the body's natural process(es). That being said, first and foremost, we promote, whenever possible, the natural healing of the body, the boosting of our bodies' immune system that fights off infection, and the importance for the body to have good nutrition in order to promote rapid healing, etc. In Western medicine medical schools, the wellness concept of 'homeostasis'—the body's tendency to monitor and maintain internal states, such as temperature and blood sugar, at fairly constant and stable levels—is a cornerstone of physiology, as homeostasis "underlies many, if not all, disease processes,"[p1] and according to Libretti and Puckett, "Diseases such as diabetes, hypertension, and atherosclerosis, involve both the disturbance of homeostasis, as well as the presence of inflammation."[2p1] The aforementioned authors explained it thusly: the body has three main types of homeostatic regulation (thermoregulation = body temperature; osmoregulation = water-to-electrolyte balance; chemical = regulates hormones, blood sugar, etc.) comprised of five primary components: stimulus (the change that 'kicks' the body out of balance); receptor (reacts to change and informs 'control unit'); control unit (communicates the change needed to bring the body back into balance); and the effector (acts on change that is needed).[2] Western medicine's healthy state of homeostasis highly values the body's own natural internal mechanisms to self-regulate and make corporal 'wellness' adjustments (in blood pressure, temperature, hormones, etc.) – without the intervention of pharmaceuticals, invasive surgery, or medical intervention(s).

In traditional healing spheres of influence, poor health, disease, misfortune (car accidents, fractures, etc.), or even unexpected successes, are not (solely) viewed as chance occurrences, but are believed to arise from the actions of individuals or ancestral spirits, according to the balance or imbalance between the individual and his/her social, spiritual, physical and/or physiological environment(s). At its core, traditional medicine can be broadly defined as "health practices, approaches, knowledge and beliefs incorporating plant, animal, and/or mineral-based medicines, spiritual therapies, manual techniques and exercises, applied singularly (or in combination) to treat, diagnose, and prevent illnesses or maintain well-being,"[3] as reported by Fokunang et al. So, we can argue that most every global region has had, at one time or another in its history, some form(s) of traditional medicine (such as Chinese, Arabic, African, Indian, etc.). These pluralistic formulas of healing are considered traditional, as they are all deeply rooted in specific socio-cultural contexts, differing from one community, or region, to another. Each region having its own unique approach to diverse health, disease, and fatalistic attitudes—even down to the level of ethno-pathogenic observations of injuries or illness. Specifically in Africa, traditional medicine "typically views sickness as the failure of complex social and spiritual relationships"; therefore it "begins diagnosis with an examination of both human and supernatural interactions".[4p2] Historically, there has also been a gross imbalance of European and American claims to global medical heritage, a narrative that oftentimes delegitimized African medical practices, agency, and contributions to global healing, provision, and treatment methodologies.[5,6]

This healthcare infrastructure accommodates both the 'generic bulk' health requirements of the 'general' public, as well as its for-profit sector competitors. Hoff's 1997 "Traditional Health Practitioners as Primary Health Care Workers"[7] study funded by the WHO, reported that incorporating trained traditional health practitioners in primary healthcare programs could be cost effective in providing essential and culturally relevant health services to communities in developing worlds. Across the globe, several surgeons, physicians, and researchers have proposed training of traditional bonesetters to reduce the incidence of gangrenous limbs, disabilities, and amputations. However, despite being consigned to a more economical, secondary placement in the health planning of developing countries, traditional (or 'indigenous') medicine practices (or more appropriately, traditional systems of health care) are gradually undergoing systemic revitalizations and rehabilitations, particularly in the last two decades.

Study Background

Our particular avenue of inquiry began in 2017 in Kumasi, Ghana, where Richter, one of the co-authors of this book, was serving as a Fulbright-Fogarty (NIH) Postdoctoral Global Health Fellow, Sub-Saharan Africa, conducting Mass-Casualty Incident (MCI) trauma research. She began investigating how to address the ever-increasing issue of fatal road traffic accidents in Ghana—as the nation progressed from a low- to middle-income country (with increasing numbers of cars, and drivers, and mass-casualty accidents). Working in collaboration with Komfe Anokye Teaching Hospital (KATH), the Kwame Nkrumah University of Technology (KNUST) was ideally located in the central and highly urbanized environs of the Ashanti Region. While there, Professor Richter (an EMT and global health professor) and Dr. Flowers (US-board certified emergency physician), observed the rather vast orthopedic ward full to the brim with young men suffering tib/fib fractures—nearly of all of whom presented with external fixators to stabilize their fractures.

One day, the co-authors went to interview a young man who had just come in with and open tib/fib fracture. When they returned the next day, they found out he had checked out 'AMA' (Against Medical Advice) to seek fracture care from a local healer/bonesetter rather than have his recommended open-fracture surgery. Both Richter and Flowers were shocked [...] Upon further enquiry they discovered that there was a troubling amount of patient mistrust surrounding Western orthopedic care. Seemingly, several patients trusted fracture treatment by traditional village "bonesetters" more than Western-trained hospital physicians. Richter and Flowers were told that oftentimes these very same patients would return to the hospital where they initially sought emergency treatment—tragically now suffering from severe gait impairments, irreversible limb deformities, life-threatening septicemia, and/or in need of a limb amputation due to gangrene—all treatable conditions that could have been prevented with appropriate healthcare. Intrigued, Richter and Flowers sought to meet, interview, and document these community care providers. However, both practitioners were keen to adopt a nonjudgmental stance throughout the interview processes in relation to the bonesetters and their past and/or current patients. Treatment strategies (massages, palpation, oral and/or topical herbal remedies, plantain-leaf bandaging, bamboo splinting, etc.) of bonesetters and patients' experiences were also examined.

Unwaveringly and unabashedly, the overriding goal for this work has never changed for us—as physicians, Emergency Medical Services (EMS) workers, surgeons, and researchers—to achieve, wherever and whenever, more efficacious and successful patient outcomes that are timely, responsive, equitable, and safe.

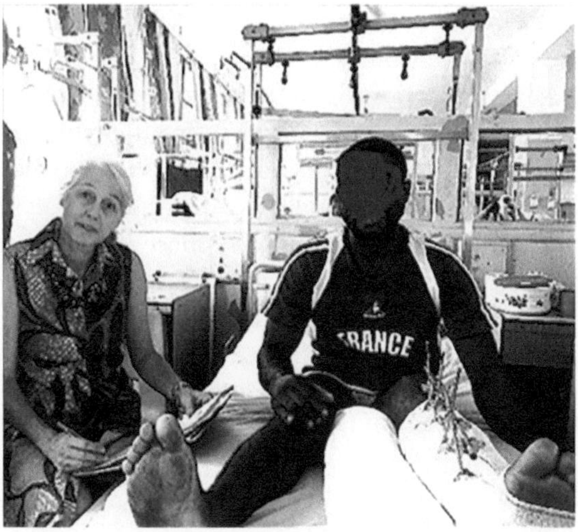

Photo 1.1. Richter interviewing orthopedic road-accident fracture patient (face obscured for privacy) about his injury management choices for Western medical care at Komfo Anokye Teaching Hospital (KATH) in Kumasi, Ghana, 2018.

With this manuscript, our intention is not to offer in-depth, exhaustive, and meticulous accounts of traditional healing practices, methodologies, ancestral remedies, and medicines within these four nations. Generally speaking, rural African treatment processes for fractures or illness usually begin with (initial) inexpensive self-treatment options, followed by traditional healing mechanisms, perhaps an expedient local pharmacy visit, followed by the final, and most costly, purview into modern Western-trained care. Wild/homegrown medicinal plants may be gainfully used at the early stages of the illness or disease at low(er) cost and, sometimes rather opportunely, can replace the indiscriminate consumption of pharmaceuticals.

Before beginning our reporting, we should note that there are inherent, built-in (and conceivably) excessive negative emphases on TBS's iatrogenic risks and outcomes of their therapies in this book (specifically) and in published research endeavors (in general). The most observable (and self-evident) bias comes from successful vs. unsuccessful fracture data accumulation, i.e., patients who have undergone successful union(s) of fractures rarely (if ever) seek a costly post-fracture 'check-up' or (ostensibly) 'superfluous' medical care at a Western biomedical facility—only those with palpable pain, evident disability, conspicuous (oftentimes malodorous) infection, and readily apparently mal-/non-union(s) will pursue more exhaustive, costly, and (potentially distressing and/or painful) medical investigations. So, inherently, there is an acknowledged bias that should be remedied via comprehensive research works that seek to collect dispassionate, balanced, and even-handed TBS biomedical patient outcomes.

As such, we have referred to three, in our opinion, particularly judicious projects: Onuminya's 2006 Nigerian study using a circumscribed collection of only one type of simple fracture—40 tibial shaft breaks[8] that allowed for a more analogous (apples-to-apples) comparative analysis. Onuminya[8] also utilized a 'control' group for a more robust scientific comparison, an important key to any proper medical investigation, and one that is rarely found in any globally published TBS treatment accounts. Another more impartial study was undertaken by the AO Alliance nonprofit in 2021 in Ghana—the Traditional Bonesetter Training Program,[9] whose goal is to prevent disabilities and complications stemming from traditional bonesetter treatments though fracture care education. The third initiative in Hawassa, Ethiopia, also supported by the AO Alliance, has created an app called BOSAD (BOne Setter Associated Disability). (For more information on these three African enquiries, see Chapter 8).

Divine and Human

We open our book with the first chapter on "Traditional Healing: The Dialectical Balance of the Divine and the Human", whereby we begin to unpack the concept of religion as an expansive tern that describes a commitment to beliefs and practices that relate to preternatural. We do not limit our understanding of African religion and healing to formal institutional dimensions of religion alone, rather what may be understood as the existence of an expansive spirituality that is always anchored in the idea of the sacred. This can be realized in many dimensions, but we engage with this in a very limited sense as all the forces around which faith and spirituality are organized. This chapter explores local cultural inferences of health, wellness, and illness and assesses how religious beliefs affect the treatment of trauma or poor health.

In our ensuing "Pathologies of Social Mechanisms" (Chapter 2), we open the discourse into how globalization, socioeconomics, and human rights have coalesced into the current diatribe between (solely) traditional and (solely) Western-based medical care access, treatment, and outcomes. Irrespective of the argument that the chasm between 'Western' medicine and 'non-European' folk/indigenous medicine is a product of post-nineteenth century medical science, the lives of millions of Africans are directly influenced by the clash(es) that continue to endure. In this chapter, the varied motivations for the usage of traditional bonesetters are analyzed. These include, but are not limited to, the following: cultural beliefs, illiteracy in human anatomy and physiology, third-party advice, a shortage of trained orthopedic specialists, fast(er), more accessible (proximity to patient) and less expensive services, fear of amputation at Western/orthodox hospitals, and poor/apathetic past experiences at hospital(s). Here we will begin the discussions of how encounters between indigenous medicine and Western medicine have been characterized by struggles, resistance, adaptation, critique, negotiation, and appropriation.

Our corresponding Chapter 3: "In Their Own Words" gives traditional bonesetters, their patients, and the orthopedic surgeons who treat TBS patients a voice. Most notably in published bonesetter research, field experts oftentimes speak ***for*** bonesetter patients, trauma surgeons, as well as the bonesetters themselves. This unique piece of literature seeks to give those actors a voice in their own words, explaining their own personal experiences in their own words. While the auspices of bonesetter practices are veiled in secrecy—locally restricted rituals, unidentified oral mixtures, secret poultice concoctions, forbidden authority, supernatural skills, exclusive privileges and birthrights, etc.—this research strives to "lift the veil" off this secretive community, and expose (both) the valuable and unsafe/dangerous practices, beliefs, and/or materials that comprise their work.

Later, in Chapter 4's "Phytochemistry, Pharmacognosy, and Ethnobotanics", we will explore (within the contexts of bone-setting practices) some natural, uncultivated, and undomesticated medicinal flora and fauna growing in Africa that have demonstrated beneficial health effects under the rigor of laboratory conditions. In this chapter, we will (to the best of our ability) review the single-most important healthcare resource for the vast majority of the world's population—wild medicinal flora and fauna. This chapter will explore a limited number of peer-reviewed studies that support the folkloric, or traditional, use of natural plant extracts, fruits, leaves, roots, flowers, and tree bark that have demonstrated potent anti-plasmodial, anti-diabetic, antimicrobial, antifungal, and other effects under laboratory conditions and phytochemical screenings.

The following chapter: "A Brief Global Overview into the Development of Orthopedic Science" looks at the history of orthopedic care, which dates back to the beginning of history itself. Regrettably, since humans first appeared on earth, they have been violently breaking bones, dislocating joints, and spraining, stretching, and tearing muscles and ligaments. There were records of treatments for orthopedic injuries that date back to the documented writings of the Egyptians, and we document the historical highlights that brought medical sciences to the heights patients enjoy today.

Chapter 6 "Back to the Basics" begins with the baseline rudimentary knowledge of a fracture, or any breach/contravention in the bone's structural continuity, with (some) degree of injury to the adjacent soft tissues. Despite the fact that there are a vast variety of fracture types (including open/compound, closed/simple, stable, unstable, transverse, oblique, spiral, etc.), some basic physiological principles in proper reduction and safe immobilization traverse across the (vast) majority of limb fractures. So, in order to proceed in an orderly investigation, it is necessary to organize our inquiry via the following general principals of the A-B-Cs of triage, trauma, reduction and immobilization, circulatory status, infection prevention, form and function, internal fixation, immobilization, complications (and how to avoid them), as well the use of imaging technologies.

In the subsequent Chapter 7, "Casualties and Complications in Fracture Management" investigates some of the primary obstacles in fracture care, such as circulation problems, management, malnutrition, patient co-morbidities, and pre-existing conditions, just to name a few. This is followed by post-TBS fracture care complications including the likes of infections, compartment syndrome, deep vein thrombosis (DVT), patella gigantism, nonunion, malunion, and more.

Taking us into today's "Current State(s) of Care," Chapter 8 delves into each nation's current inflation rates, healthcare expenditures, GDP per capita, purchasing power, and median income—and how those affect each nation's orthopedic care competencies and capacities—or lack thereof. We will review access and availability challenges of imaging diagnostics, specialized surgeons, instrumentation, as well as new African NGOs and programs that are attempting to 'close the gap' between affordable and dependable musculoskeletal injury care. We also review how expensive 'big-ticket' orthopedic surgical instrumentation and implants invariably 'out-price' average patients in sub-Saharan Africa and other Low- and Middle- Income Countries (LMICs) across the globe.

In Chapter 9, the authors set out on a path to constructively assemble a veritable "How-To" guide on moving traditional bone-setting practitioners and their practices into safer protocols and practices throughout mainstream African healthcare infrastructures. With a generous list of 28 recommendations, the authors seek to map out clear-cut and cost-effective mechanisms for sub-Saharan African nations to safely and successfully identify, motivate, train, and incorporate TBS into their current healthcare infrastructures. The 28 recommendations include simple bone fracture protocol algorithms, user-friendly TBS iPhone apps, web-based platforms, herb-drug interaction assessments, government and Ministry of Health mandates, post-fracture physical therapy guidance, and much, much more.

Finally, Chapter 10 "Facing Forward" discourse ends our study with an optimistic, forward-looking vision of the Human Right to Health, one that recognizes the right of everyone to enjoy the highest attainable standard of physical and mental health—all in congruous alignment toward our aim of efficacious patient outcomes that are timely, responsive, equitable, and safe.

ACKNOWLEDGMENTS

Throughout this nine-year study, we have had many hospitals, universities, physicians, orthopedic surgeons, professors, and university students to thank. We are indebted to Richter's former Kwame Nkrumah University of Science and Technology student, Ebenezer Owusu-Sekyere, who introduced us to the three bonesetters that were interviewed in remote areas surrounding Kumasi, Ghana. Ebenezer spoke to the traditional bonesetters, explaining our motivations, and served as our translator for each of the interviews. We also want to thank Wellington Mukumba, a native of Zimbabwe, for helping locate, translate, and get information on our two Zimbabwean bonesetters. We also wish to thank: Komfo Anokye Teaching Hospital (Kumasi, Ghana); Kwame Nkrumah University of Science and Technology's (Kumasi, Ghana) Vice Dean of the School of Medical Sciences, Professor Faye; and the University of Gondar's (Gondar, Ethiopia) School of Medical Sciences.

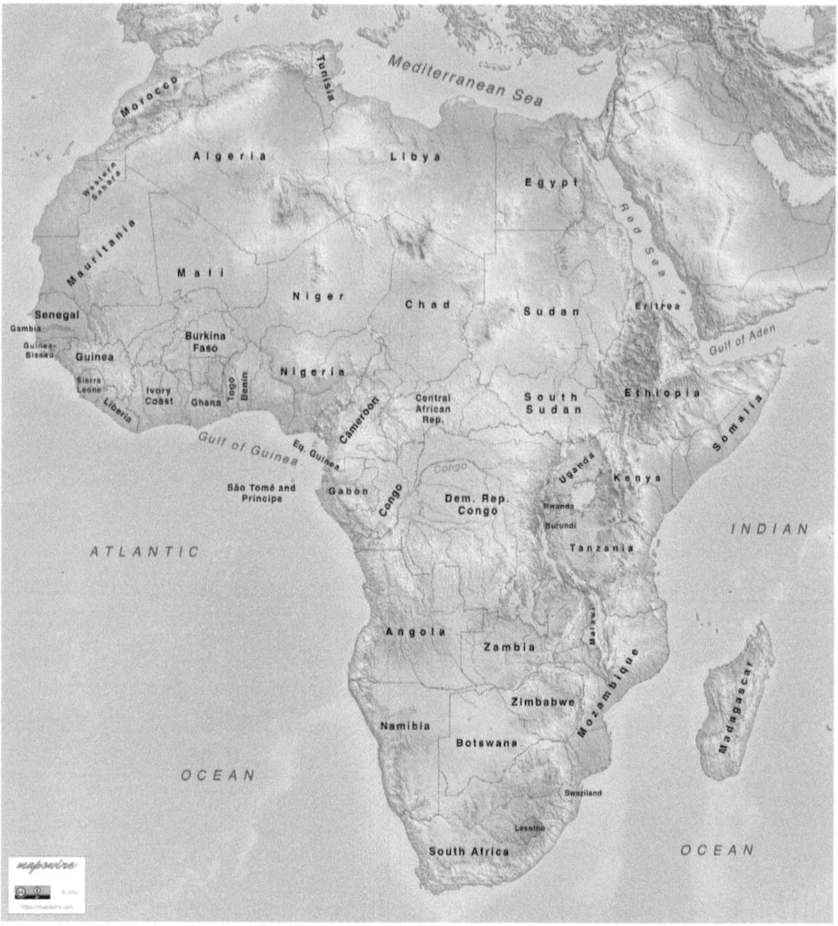

Figure 1.1. Map of Africa indicating the general primary global locations of the four traditional medicine bonesetters' countries studied: Ghana (west Africa); Cameroon (central Africa); Ethiopia (east Africa, Horn of Africa); and Zimbabwe (south Africa). Copyright: Mapswire, 2022.

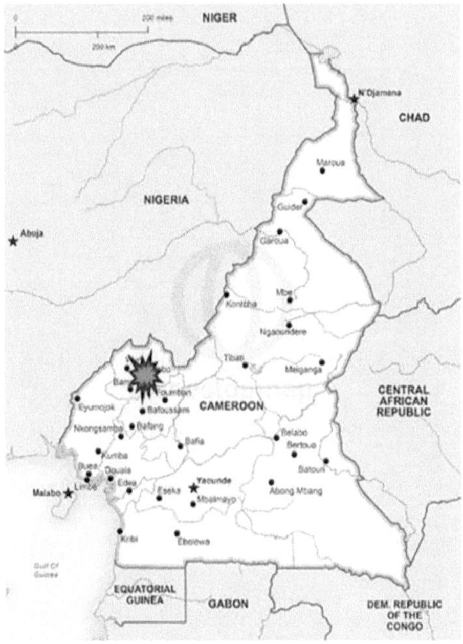

Figure 1.2. Map of Cameroon indicating the main location of the studied bonesetter region in the Donga Mantung administrative district. Copyright: onestopmap.com, 2023.

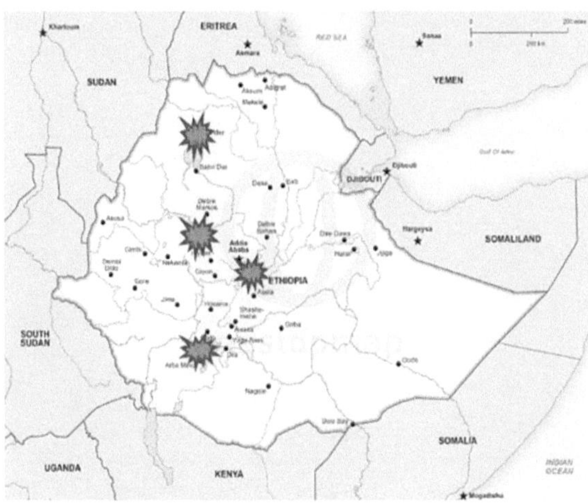

Figure 1.3. Map of Ethiopia indicating a few of the research sites, like the University of Gondar Teaching Hospital (Gondar); Wolaita Sodo (southern region); Debra Markos Hospital (East Gojjam); Arbo Minch (Gamo zone); Tikur Anbessa specialized hospital; and Black Lion Teaching Hospital in Addis Ababa. Copyright: onestopmap.com, 2023.

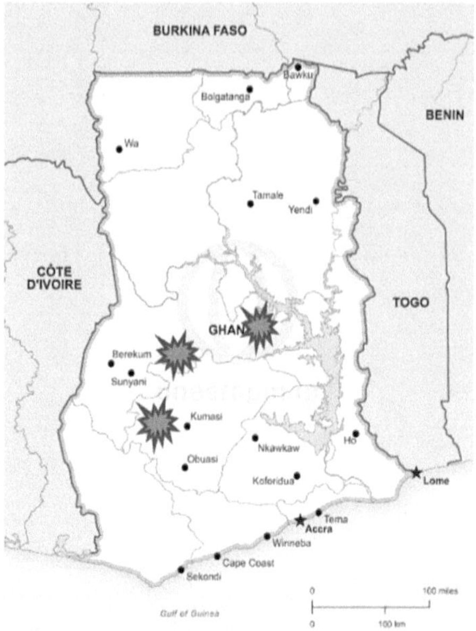

Figure 1.4. Map of Ghana indicating the main locations of the studied bonesetter region(s), including Akumsa Dumase and Kumasi. Copyright: onestopmap.com, 2023.

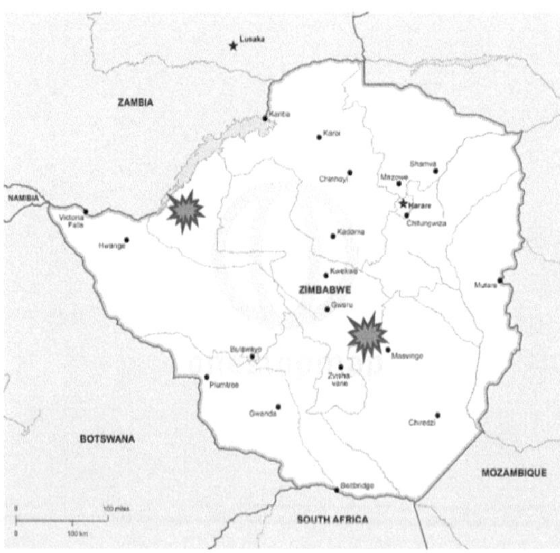

Figure 1.5. Map of Zimbabwe indicating the main locations of the studied bonesetter region(s), specifically the Masvingo Province (southeast of Harare), and Midlands Province (Gokwe Nembudziya), bordering Zambia to the northwest. Copyright: onestopmap.com, 2023.

ABOUT THE AUTHORS

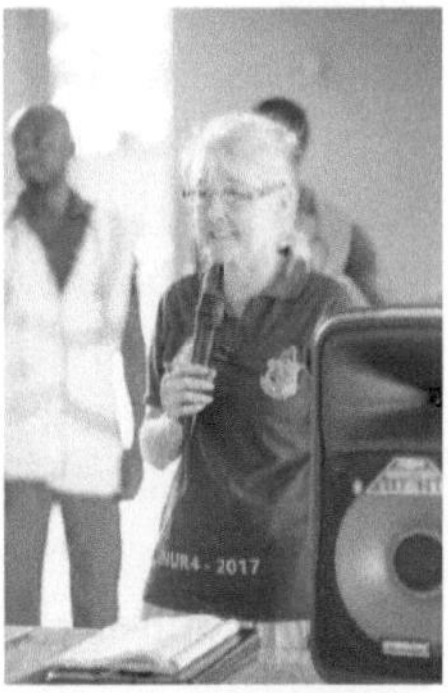

Roxane E. Richter, Ph.D. E.M.T., is an Assistant Professor, School of Public Health, University of Louisville. She has been distinguished as a Fulbright Specialist in Medical Mass Casualty Planning & Response (Ghana), U.S. Embassy Ambassador Distinguished Scholar (University of Gondar, Ethiopia), and a Fulbright-Fogarty NIH Postdoctoral Global Health Fellow (Sub-Saharan Africa). She received her doctorate from the University of the Witwatersrand in Johannesburg, South Africa. Her four decades of humanitarian aid service (American Red Cross Disaster Health Services, World Missions Possible, House of Charity, Rotary Int., United Methodist Church, Yonkofa Project, etc.), and her professional research focuses on advancing prehospital patient injury/trauma care, vision care, and disaster/Mass Casualty Incident planning, and preparedness in sub-Saharan Africa. She served on international emergency medical care teams to Ethiopia, South Africa, Swaziland, Zambia, Togo, Sierra Leone, USA, and Ghana. She has been honored as a crowned Queen Mother (*Ohemaa Ama Oyamyiefo*: "Saturday-Born Queen Mother of Compassion") in Ekumfi Ekotsi-Bogyano, Ghana. She is a published author of numerous articles, and her books include: "Medical Outcasts: Gendered and Institutionalized Xenophobia in Undocumented Forced Migrants' Emergency Health Care" and "Witchcraft as a Social Diagnosis: Traditional Ghanaian Beliefs and Global Health". She has traveled to 75 nations and her future goals are to further develop her 'A-E-M-S' MCI algorithm, 'Gender-Aware Disaster Care' programs, and other innovations in prehospital trauma care in low-resource healthcare systems.

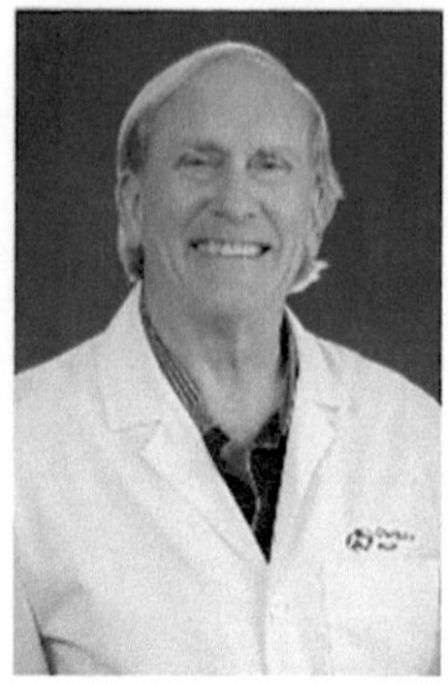

Dr. Thomas M. Flowers is a certified emergency physician with the American Board of Emergency Medicine since 1992. He currently practices at the Family Community Clinic in Saipan, Northern Marianas Island. He was recently recognized by the American Board of Emergency Medicine for holding 30 consecutive years of certification as a Board-Certified physician. He has been an Advanced Cardiac Life Support instructor for over 10 years and is also trained in Advanced wound care and Hyperbaric Medicine. He has practiced in emergency medicine in Texas, Kentucky, Arizona, the United Kingdom, and New Zealand. Through various nonprofits (Rotary International, World Missions Possible, United Methodist Church) Dr. Flowers has taught EMS coursework, led, and served on international medical care teams to Ethiopia, South Africa, Swaziland, Zambia, Togo, Sierra Leone, USA, and Ghana. He is a published author of several medical sciences articles, and a co-author of the 2017 book: "Witchcraft as a Social Diagnosis: Traditional Ghanaian Beliefs and Global Health" published by Lexington Books. He is the current Medical Director of World Missions Possible, a 501c3 nonprofit www.worldmissionspossible.org.

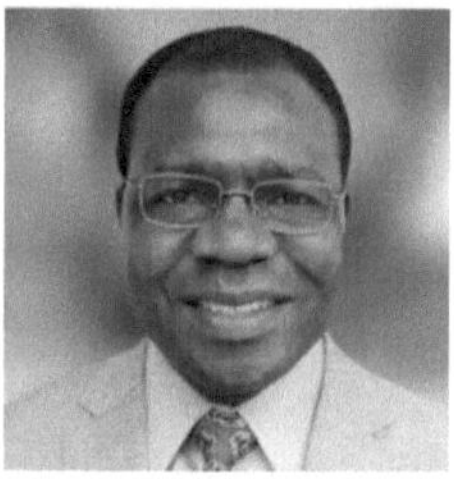

Elias K. Bongmba, Ph.D., is a tenured Professor of Religion at Rice University in Houston, Texas; Harry & Hazel Chavanne Chair in Christian Theology; Professor of Religion, Faculty Assoc. Wiess College; President of the African Assoc. for the Study of Religion; recipient of the 2020 Ray L. Hart Service Award from the American Academy of Religion. A native of Cameroon, he combines his teaching of African religions and his research in theology and philosophy of religion working with African philosophical ideas and Continental philosophy. He is author of four books, three edited books, and has authored 60 peer reviewed essays and book chapters. His books include: "African Witchcraft and Otherness: A Philosophical and Theological Critique of Intersubjective Relations"; "The Dialectics of Transformation in Africa" (which won the 2007 Franz Fanon Prize for outstanding work in Caribbean Thought, "Facing a Pandemic: The African Church and the Crisis of AIDS", and "Witchcraft as Social Diagnosis: Traditional Ghanaian Beliefs and Global Health". He is editor of The Wiley Blackwell Companion to African Religions, (Malden, Mass: Wile Blackwell, 2012) and The Rutledge Companion to Christianity in Africa, (New York: Routledge, 2015). He is also Co-Editor of Living on the Edge: Essays in Honour of Steve de Gruchy Activist & Theologian, eds. James R. Cochrane, Elias Bongmba, Isabel Phiri, Des van der Water. (Pietermaritzburg, South Africa: Cluster Publications, 2012).

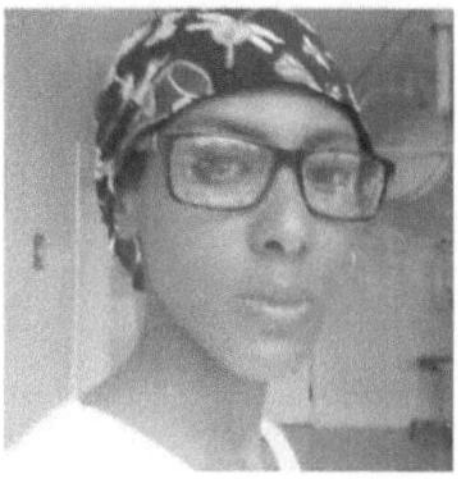

Dr. Ananya K. Admasu is an Assistant professor in Orthopedics, FCS (Ortho) ECSA. Dr. Admasu is an Assistant Professor in Orthopedics Lecturer, Orthopedic and Trauma Consultant College of Medicine and Health Sciences at the University of Gondar, Ethiopia. She also works as an Orthopedic Sales Consultant for Zimmer Biomet (total hip and knee replacement procedures), and Ortimplant-Turkey (complex trauma procedures). In 2019, she established the first Orthopedics department and launched a residency program at the University of Gondar—only 1 of 7 Orthopedic training programs in Ethiopia at that time. She also was the head of the Orthopedics and traumatology department at the University of Gondar (2019–2021), managing the planning, budgeting, and supervision of both clinical and academic departments. She remains an active global surgery advocate as a SURGhub Ambassador; founder of Female Orthopedic Empowerment Program (FOEP) and Tenaye.com; and the host of "The Everyday Leader with Dr. Ananya" podcast.

DECLARATION OF PATIENT CONSENT

The authors certify that they have obtained all appropriate patient consent forms translated (verbally and written) in various languages. In the form the patient(s) has/have given his/her/their consent for his/her/their images and other clinical information to be reported in the journal. The patients understand that their names and initials will not be published and due efforts will be made to conceal their identity, but anonymity cannot be guaranteed.

Financial support and sponsorship

None.

CONFLICTS OF INTEREST

There are no conflicts of interest.

Chapter 1

TRADITIONAL HEALING: THE DIALECTICAL BALANCE OF THE DIVINE AND THE HUMAN

We begin this study with a cursory observation that healing (in some of the African contexts we are familiar with) call for a holistic perspective—as healing and wellbeing in many African communities embraces spiritual dimensions (anchored in the idea of the sacred), but which we employ as all the forces around which faith and spirituality are organized. Our study is limited to a quest to understand one dimension of fracture healing by bone-setting practitioners as 'traditional healers'. It is not our intent to offer a fully developed study of African medical traditions; rather, we focus narrowly on the treatment of bone fractures provided by local healers who learned their medical practices from family members or other caregivers, rather than through Westernized biomedical curricula.

A second distinction is important, namely that we do not pursue causative relationships between religion and healing within the confines of this book. Nonetheless, we neither disregard nor eschew any (or all) relationship(s) between religion and healing. And as our research continued over the years, it became more and more clear to us that religious dimensions of traditional bone-setting could not be ignored. Indeed, several studies from Africa demonstrate a resilient, intense, and intricate relationship between religion and healing. For example, in the study by Fokunang et al.,[3] we see that Western biomedical treatment "is divorced from the patient's culture; family and community," and, "Patients are removed from the family and community, stripped of their identity and forced into a sterile hospital setting," and that the treatment "only addresses a patient's biological manifestation of the illness and does not attempt to heal spiritual aspects of illness."[p285] This is the place and the role of traditional medical practitioners, in stark contrast with Western medicine, which is based in technical and analytical evidence-based, peer-reviewed research.

Largely, the explosion of local traditional therapies in different parts of Africa has been attributed to a dearth of affordable and accessible healthcare systems (particularly, in rural areas), forcing local people to treat themselves via cost-free wild medicinal plants or cheap roadside remedies (that predispose patients to unknown, unregulated, and/or unsafe ingredients). Generally speaking, the vast majority of African patients begin their healing journeys via self-treatment (prior to a visit to a traditional healer, pharmacist, or a modern hospital- or clinic-based doctor). Wild medicinal plants are used at an early stage of the illness, conveniently, and cost-effectively replacing indiscriminate consumption of drugs purchased from pharmacies (usually distributed without a physician's prescription, government testing oversight, adverse side-effect monitoring, drug/food interaction investigations, and even substandard/falsified ingredients).

Recent studies indicate that despite the fact that Africans have known medical services offered by Colonial and Post-Colonial governments and religious-based medical work—Africa's quest for traditional healing remains strong. A recent 2025 study by Juliet Amarachukwwu Nwafor, Roland Edet, and Ezebunwa Nwokocha demonstrates that after several decades of missionary medicine and other forms of biomedical interventions in Africa, people still seek medical help from the practitioners of indigenous of local medicine.[10] After mapping the complexity of Lagos, Nigeria, a city teeming with immigrants, the aforementioned authors argue specifically that many people in the city still prefer to seek out medical remedies from traditional healers.[10] The authors also stated that one of the lessons that should be gleaned from the Lagos' public routine is "the need for targeted public health interventions, including culturally sensitive healthcare programs, improved sanitation and expanded access to affordable healthcare services."[10]

Somehow, as academics, healthcare practitioners, and researchers, we continue to take it for granted that religion *has* played an important role in wellness, healing, and health—and *will* continue to do so into our foreseeable future. While we respect the distinctions between religion as faith, cultural, and shared social practice(s), biomedical healing practices involve scientific research engagements, common theoretical knowledge, and high-tech processes. We want to note that copious innumerable scientific mechanisms involved in biomedicine—even traditional medicine in the African context—has not distanced itself (too) far from the idea, or the practices, of religion.

Idea of the Sacred

We must also point out that the concept of religion is an expansive term that describes a commitment to beliefs and practices that relate to preternatural. We do not limit our understanding of religion and healing to formal institutional dimensions of religion alone, rather what may be understood as the existence of an expansive spirituality that is always anchored in the idea of the sacred. Tanzanian theologian Laurenti Magesa offers inimitable perspectives on the historical and daily impact of religion on the lives of many people across Africa via two studies, his 2013 book entitled What is Not Sacred? African Spirituality,[11] and in his 1997 book entitled African Religion: The Moral Traditions of the Abundant Life.[12] The construct of religion includes an understanding and affirmation of the role religion plays in health and wellbeing that are still attributed to spiritual beings (regardless of scientific knowledge on disease causation), or ancestors that cause illness or initiate misfortune due to a lack of ancestral offerings, libation, and/or ancestral veneration.[11,12] Family members often call on ancestors to positively intervene when they are faced with illness, and pay their respects to ancestors (solely) in the hopes of regaining their health.

Religion, Tradition and Healing

What we consider the complex (and contested) relationship between religion and healing is now an established twentieth-century 'Revelation'. While this book is not focused on religion and healing *per se*, it is still important that we briefly highlight the intersections that exist between religion and bone-fracture treatment (without revisiting nineteenth-century religion and healing interpretations). In this manuscript, we use religion (in general) to refer to those practices by individuals or groups, which relate humans to higher spiritual force(s) that are seen by their followers as either the source (or sustainer) of human existence. While religious organizations are also not the focus of this study, we would be remiss not to state that religion as an institution and praxis has influenced, perhaps disproportionately, the understanding of illness and misfortunes (some consider fracture as a misfortune) for many communities in the African context, as well as in many other global contexts.

It is quite customary in many places in Africa to hear people discuss illness in relationship to religion; in those discussions, religion is often seen as a viable resource for coping, treating, and/or combating the illness. As one example, the Wimbum people of the northwest region of Cameroon, people often talk about "*yang Nyu*" (which literally translates to "God's illness"), but is conversely, inferred to be understood as a 'natural' illness. Fractures, much like disease and illnesses, are identified and characterized by not just one, but several, differing respects and disciplines. If someone suffers a broken bone, it can be acknowledged as an accident or misfortune—or a diviner may be consulted if the patient suspected that the misfortune was 'caused' by someone who placed a curse on them. We should point out that amongst the Zimbabwean Shona people, as well as other African communities, there is a recognition that some ethereal spirits are problematic via the 'unleashing' of human misfortune(s). And while good spirits bring good health and beneficial advice to bonesetters on healing fractures—evil spirits are dynamic, powerful agents of misfortune. In saying this, we do not claim that relatives or friends do not directly inquire about causation—as one of the common expressions used in the Wimbum area in Cameroon, instructs that: "*There must have been something.*" In the Wimbum community, whenever someone uses that expression, they are making a claim that an illness or misfortune was, in fact, not a natural occurrence, but rather caused by evil forces or witchcraft. However, it is much more likely at the present time, according to Bongmba, for the victim to spend their money on traditional healers or hospital stays rather than spending large sums of money on ritual specialist(s) who would claim to reveal the evildoer. For Ethiopians, who take great national pride in being considered 'religious', according to Admasu, the patient's choice of a religious healer or healing method are extremely critical factors when choosing their care provider(s). Indeed, according to Pew Research Center, some 78% of Ethiopians attend church weekly, 65% claim to pray daily (65%), and nearly all (98%) say religion is "very important" in their lives (compared that to 6% of Orthodox Christian Russians and 52% of Americans).[13]

Divine Healers

Indigenous healing encompasses the religious '*Weltanschauung*' of the healer, so it irresoluble to characterize a 'typical African healer', as there are many types, and the cultural diversity and complexity of their practices are encyclopedic when considered in detail. We simply cannot offer a singular, one-dimensional description or clarification of the African men and women who practice traditional bone-setting. Many of them (like Pa Tamnjong, who will be introduced later) admit patients into their private household compounds, so the therapeutic environment is one of a close social and familial engagement, whereby the patient lives with the family of the traditional healer. However, one trait that Cameroonian healers seemingly have in common, according to Bongmba, is that they describe and explain illness in terms of social interaction and that they act on the belief that religion permeates every aspect of human existence. We further agree that a very important aspect of traditional treatment is that some of the traditional healers foster a deep personal relationship with the patient, and that the 'social' aspects of the therapeutic process require reciprocity. Here we must point out, as Fokunang et al. does, that "the magical inclination of Cameroonian traditional medicine takes nothing away from the fact that some of the healers now are experienced and skilled in biomedical components of their profession."[3] And while we cannot definitively address all the religious dimension(s) of bone-setting practices, we note the observations from Alegbeleye regarding their study of bone-setting (Kumbo-Nso in the Bui Division of Cameroon)[14] that the practice is patronized by clients who belong to differing religions. Alegbelye's 2019 study demonstrates that most of the practitioners claimed that they inherited the practice from supernatural force(s)—some type of divine lifeforce, mystical power, and/or bygone ancestor who had passed the trade knowledge to a descendant of their family.[14]

In many parts of Africa, the view that God or divine beings show healers how to manage certain illnesses or fractures was a common theme employed by healers. For example, one 1904 study conducted and published by J. Graham Forbes in the Gold Coast demonstrated that treating fractures was not practiced in some regions of West Africa.[15] He argued that while local medical practice handled other illnesses, they did not treat fractures[15]:

> Fractures are as a rule left untreated; in the case of a fractured phalanx, the finger may be amputated. One native whom I saw in the forest suffered from an ununited fracture of the right humerus, the result of a blow from a falling branch fifteen years before. The only treatment he received from a native 'doctor' was the application of pieces of wood to the arm for three days, smeared with some herb preparation, after which nothing further was done. The flail-like limb could only be raised to the level of the shoulder, and apparently a false joint had formed between the ununited ends of the bone. The case of a boy whom I saw in a northern village was, fortunately for him, treated differently. Two months previously he had sustained a fracture of the right femur. When I saw him, he was lying on the ground of the hut with the right leg partially embedded in a trough dug in the earth, and fixed in position with pegs driven in on each side. Firm union had resulted without shortening of the limb, and soon after he was at work again in the fields.[p362]

In another study, Mbih Jerome Tosam has underscored the religious dimension of healing in some African contexts, arguing that "traditional African medicine… and healthcare are established on beliefs, values, and customs that are linked to a deeply spiritual and holistic worldview."[16p255] In the village of Ntumbaw in the Donga Mantung Division of the northwest region of Cameroon, religion was (and remains) a central part of the lives of the people of Ntumbaw, as well as in the mentioned Njirong, Ngulu, and Sop Villages. The two main religions in this area are Christianity

(Berean Baptist Church in Ntumbaw, Baptist Church in Njirong, Saint Martin de Porres Catholic Church of Ntumbaw) and Islam (Donga Mantung Division, drawing many of its members from the Hausa and Fulani people).

Studies from different parts of Africa indicate that faith communities have also expanded their healthcare services, which undoubtably impact African religious healings' resonances. Some examples include the Association of Church-Based Development Projects (ACDEP at https://acdep.org) Traditional Medicine Project, and the Ghana Traditional and Alternative Medicine Directorate that uses radio commercials to motivate healers to join its organization and network with public health managers (for more information, see Chapter 9, Recommendation #16). These studies, in our view, shine a spotlight on the considerable attempts to promote pluralism via African medicine.

Why Religion?

Academic studies of healing (in relationship to religion) is an established discipline that offers numerous resources to interdisciplinary scholars working in the field of religion, health, sociology, medicine, ethnobotanicals, philosophy, and African Studies. When seeking an understanding of Africa's health challenges, why is religion important? In Koening et al.'s second edition of the massive 2012 "Handbook of Religion and Health", the editors and their collaborators offer a rich and detailed account of the relationship that exists between religion and healing—pointing out that a search for the title religion and health yielded a stunning 152,000 hits.[17] So why is there such an ongoing fascination between the intersections of religion and health? The researchers argue that there is growing interest in the field and their work offers a historical account of the relationship between the two disciplines, defining the different subfields of the discipline (such as spirituality), or even terms that are related (like secular humanism). But most importantly, their work offers scholars a detailed mapping of the exhaustive and compelling research that has been accomplished in religion and health.

Songs of Healing

Janzen's 1992 book "Discourses of Healing in Central Africa"[18] offers a broader and more expansive study of therapeutic traditions in the central and southern African regions. These therapeutic practices addressed different states of health and spiritual contexts ranging from the role and place of spirits in illness. The strength of this study lies in the fact that

Janzen captured the employment of this therapeutic practice in several countries in the region. Thus, readers were introduced into how important a role 'performance' can play in healing. Janzen's interpretation of '*ngoma*' (rituals or celebrations that use drumming, dance, and song) made a case for how song and drumming were part of healing practices in the region.[18] He began with a straightforward affirmation that discourse is central to the construction of knowledge about misfortune and healing. The author also offers historical, cultural, (and in our view) dynamic accounts and analyses of illness and therapy in central and Southern Africa that take a number of forms—the evocation of distress and hope before others, prayers to God, ancestors, and spirits.[18]

Ancestral Interventions

Other studies of religion and healing have given readers targeted local insights that demonstrate the breadth of the long practice(s) of traditional healing that are grounded in local religious cultures. For example, Zimbabwean scholars of religion carried out a study of Shona healing ministries as practiced by practitioners of Zimbabwean indigenous religions. The healing ministries of African churches in Zimbabwe reported to believe in different spirits and that particular ancestral spirits can (and do) cause illness.[19] These inflicted ailments could defy and outmaneuver human treatment—but not kill the patient—as the illness was to remind the person of their ancestorial obligations to the spiritual ancestor and their society. We make this point as in some African thought, ancestors are treated as exceptional persons who have died, and who continue to provide support for relatives; in turn, those mortal relatives are expected to respect their immortal ancestors, and follow the set moral and cultural examples they established when they were alive.

In some ways, we could make a case that there are strong religious dimensions to some bone-setting practices—strictly based on the grounds that skills are passed on from ancestors to the current practitioner. Ancestors are seen as spiritual beings in some African communities, rife with the power to bestow blessings, great fortunes, and wellbeing. Family members will devote huge amounts of time, expense, and consideration to their ancestors by dedicating lavish offerings and costly libations in their honor. The sacredness of ancestral practices in Africa has been well documented, as they have never been completely decimated (despite the Pentecostal revolution's attempts to scientifically dominate and demean practices). Therefore, it is safe to argue that whether acknowledged or unacknowledged, beliefs will always play a role in religious healing rituals.

Cultural Influence

Recognition of local cultural inferences of health, wellness, and illness is paramount when assessing how religious beliefs affect the treatment of trauma or poor health. For example, in Richter's (2015) book entitled "Medical Outcasts," the studied group of Zimbabwean Shona women seeking emergency healthcare in South Africa discerned no direct correlation between somatic symptoms and their emotional health.[20] Physical complaints among the Shona population, especially those concerning the head or heart corporal areas, were more so considered 'manifestations' of cultural metaphors that could be readily dismissed as "thinking too much" (known as '*kufungisisa*') during times of stress.[20]

We mention this as beliefs weigh heavily on the religious and medical orientation(s) on the lives within an African community. In this sense, we can view religion as a praxis that is embedded in the broad(er) cultural system, in which the idea (and state) of wellbeing adopts religious dimensions. We take this position in that our 'holistic perspective' embraces communities, individual healers, and other cultural specialists in order to form a broader perspective of social, spiritual, cultural, and even local political dimensions (when indigenous African leaders like kings, queens, and chiefs act as health advocates in their communities). This leads us to state that studies like this demonstrate that many people in African communities continue to see medical interventions through a *bricolage* that envisions divine forces, ancestors, medical interventions offered by biomedical experts, traditional doctors, and/or native healers. The services and practices in which local health experts, often described as traditional doctors or healers, offer continue to play a meaningful role in African communities.

Another authoritative source book on African religion and healing is the formidable reference is the work edited by John Gray entitled "Ashe, Traditional Religion and Healing in Sub-Saharan Africa and the Diaspora: A Classified International Bibliography."[21] However, Janzen's classic book "The Quest for Therapy: Medical Pluralism in Lower Zaire", is a rich text, in which Janzen demonstrates the social and spiritual (otherworldly) dimensions of healing.[22] The study focused and articulated the understanding of illness and the search for solutions within social communal, spiritual, and pluralistic spheres (where illness and misfortunes are addressed via therapeutic systems). The study highlighted the significant role played in the understanding and treatment of ailments by the '*nganga*' (Shona healer), who acknowledged their patient-care limitations by referring acutely ill patients to local area hospitals.[22] Studies by Michael Gelfand among the Shona people of Zimbabwe pointed to the religious and spiritual dimension of the medical work done by the a '*nganga*' whose medical work is intrinsically tied to spiritual leadership.[23] Gelfand portrayed the '*nganga*' as a healer who treats people with herbs and "advises the people or patients on the methods and procedure of propitiation and other rituals in order to stop the cause [...] Thus [the *nganga* medical practice] is 'partly spiritual and partly homeopathic'."[23p25]

In the Postcolonial Era

The Cameroon government, as well as Cameroonians, in the postcolonial era remained concerned about indigenous health systems, and oftentimes championed the work that was done by local healers. Our co-author Bongmba recalls that in the Njirong and Ntumbaw villages there were several traditional healers who had a wide reputation in the northwest region of Cameroon. In the past, traditional healers were identified by various titles including: herbalist, traditional healers, native doctors, and (in older literature) as 'witch doctors', a derogatory term that ignored the broad spiritual, material, social, and financial transactions involved in these age-old African medical practices. Beginning in the late 1950s, traditional medical practices boomed in Cameroon. In the Donga Mantung administrative district in Cameroon (where Bongmba grew up), the government established a main district hospital at Nkambe, and later on in Ndu Sub-District and other sub-districts as part of the policy of the Ministry of Public Health to make health services more readily accessible. Additionally, faith-based organizations in Cameroon continued to manage many hospitals that they had established as part of their missionary and humanitarian work. In the late sixties, most of the seventies, and early 1980s, medical services offered by traditional Cameroonian herbalists was going through what may be described as a rebirth, or resurgence. To be sure, Cameroon was not a complete healthcare desert during that time period, as the system was managed by the government of Cameroon through its Ministry of Public Health, including provincial, divisional, and in many cases, sub-divisional hospitals.

The resurgence in the demand for these herbal therapies increased when Cameroon faced an acute economic crisis in the 1980s (shocking many in vast oil-producing country); this was an economic crisis that Cameroon and other countries faced when the World Bank and the International Monetary Fund imposed their Structural Adjustment Program (fiscal austerity, liberalization of trade policies, economic privatization, etc.). In an effort to provide some economic relief, the government of Cameroon (in collaboration with the WHO) promoted the use of herbal medicines, and more importantly, worked to bring the use of free and/or low-cost traditional medicines into the healthcare infrastructure.

In 1981, the Cameroon government, under the leadership of (then) President Ahmadu Ahidjo, articulated proposals to integrate traditional medicine into the nation's health infrastructure. Since then, traditional medicine has been recognized (but not regulated), gleaning community respect and value as they offer medical care in underserved and unreached areas. This move by the government of Cameroon brought enormous visibility to traditional doctors, and more notably, elevated and thrust traditional medicine up and into the spheres of national health plans.

During this resurgence, the government of Cameroon worked with local and international researchers that had previously demonstrated interest in traditional medicine, and worked with stakeholders to create responsible associations to promote research and critical dialogue. There was little societal pushback against this move, as even physicians and professors at the University of Yaoundé Medical School recognized traditional medicine's public appeal. It is important to note here that when the other universities in Cameroon started their own medical schools, professors had, at the time, also expressed an interest in traditional medicine, according to Bongmba. In our opinion, it remains an area where continued scientific research and strict monitoring services could and should ensure best practices to strengthen the integration of traditional ethnobotanicals into national healthcare systems. Initially, it was believed that such integration was to be completed sometime after 2012 in Cameroon.[271] In collaboration with the WHO, a plan was put in place to provided institutional support for the work that traditional healers do, according to Bongmba, to promote the cultivation of beneficial medicinal plant species, as well as the employment of adequate technologies that would promote, protect, and regulate sustainable ecological harvesting of natural resources (as opposed to rampant, unsustainable over-harvesting). All of these developments in Cameroon were to be implemented as part of the United Nation's global Millennium Development Goals (MDGs) in order to reduce poverty, morbidity, and mortality, while supporting more sustainable healthcare developments.

In 2019, Alegbelye published a very insightful study of bone-setting practices in northwest Cameroon. Alegbelye carried out his research when he was affiliated with the Shisong Catholic Hospital (Bui Division), noting that these TBS services were not only popular, desired, and patronized by patients, but also complicated, challenging, and costly.[14] Alefbeleye and his co-authors pointed out that the government of Cameroon had offered a strategic platform to promote traditional medical practices, and that the nation was an optimal designation due to its significant diversity of flora and fauna.[14] This rich biological biodiversity is associated with the diversity of the ethnic groups, reports Alegbeleye et al., in which each "contributes a unique ethno-pharmacopoeia and to Cameroon a national therapeutic patrimony, which is the richest in Africa."[14p285] Alegbeleye et al. argued that "the limited scientific evidence about TM/CAM's safety and efficacy as well as other considerations make it important for governments to step into the TM practice, research and development within the frame work of integration into the primary, communal and national health care system in Cameroon."[14p85]

Nkongmeneck et al. added that "since the 90's the fields of study have expanded to include ethno-pharmacology, phytochemistry, chemistry of natural products, organic synthesis and the usefulness of medicinal and aromatic plants."[24p24] Unfortunately, due to widespread state-interest research, carried out at universities, and the promotion of these research activities by the Ministry of Research and Innovation, some medicinal plants (especially anti-Malarial compounds) suffered the adverse impacts of abusive over-harvesting.

Folklore of the Boa Bonesetter of Cameroon, Pa Tamnjong

As we've mentioned before, it is difficult to typify a Cameroonian healer, as there are diverse types, and the cultural diversity and complexity of their practices are encyclopedic, when considered in detail. Perhaps some traits most Cameroonian traditional healers have in common is that they rationalize illness via social interaction(s), and they act on the belief that religion permeates every aspect of human existence, according to Bongmba. As one example, a traditional healer who specialized in treating bone fractures in Ntumbaw Village was Pa Tamnjong, who was a member of the Shokop sub-chiefdom in Ntumbaw Village. The authors have been granted the use of his true name (and all other bonesetters in this book) as a way of recognizing their medical practices. Bongmba interviewed Tamnjong and family members first in the late 1990s. Pa Tamnjong was known to be a very simple, yet personable, individual. His name Tamnjong is an indication that he was a member of the Manjong society, and he carried a leadership rank in that society. The Manjong society (along with the Nfu society) are sociocultural monikers, but also considered the two military organizations in Wimbum Village (these two societies are designated as 'decision-makers' in times of war).

When Bongmba arrived in the village to interview Pa Tamnjong, he had just recently retired from his healing practices. With the help of his many assistants, he described in very basic terms that his work was "a gift from God". He carried out the treatment of fractures in his compound. In cases where he determined that the fracture was acute, the patient was encouraged to stay with him as long as it was necessary to fully heal. He charged a modest amount for his treatment and accepted payment in cash or in livestock (usually goats or sheep, or a guineafowl for minor injuries). The aged bonesetter described his appeal to the profession by saying he used his gift to help people with their injuries. At the time, he indicated that he had not lost one patient. He had seen difficult fractures (in which the leg—literally—hung in the balance, so to speak), but he reiterated that in such a situation he continued to treat the patient and depend on the power of God to make the medicine and the treatment work. One thing Pa Tamnjong admitted was the fact that the profession he had chosen was exceptionally demanding. Some of the patients lived with him for a long time. In some cases, the patient's relatives also stayed at Pa Tamnjong's healing center. Nonetheless, in a society where hospitality is an all-important virtue, quantifying the real cost of such long-term housing and treatment is incalculable, so Pa believed this was all part and parcel of his "God-given mission".

The public at large claimed he also had very strong mystical powers. It was alleged that when patient came for treatment, Pa Tamnjong would receive the patient and relax them. Pa Tamnjong would ask the patient to wait for him, stay calm, and not worry if he saw anything. He would caution the patient to remain seated. Pa Tamnjong would then go to a nearby lake about a half of a mile away (that was believed to be a sacred space) and incarnate into a boa constrictor. The boa constrictor would come to the house, lick the fracture, and wrap itself around the fracture, adjusting itself in order to bring the bones together. Then Pa Tamnjong would return and begin the physical treatment using specifically designed tools to hold the fracture together, and to apply his homemade remedies on the fracture. Much of this account had a spiritually powerful dimension to it, as well as local lore. The role of the viper adds not only mystique, but points to a mystical practice enhanced by the physicality of a powerful animal.

Religion vs. Science?

Studies demonstrate that there is a strong relationship between religion and science. Elaine Ecklund has argued that the idea that religious people ignore science is simply not true.[25] Thus, we cannot entertain the view that religion has nothing to do within the complexities of the physiological healing processes. As one example, in a 2023 study carried out in Japan, Daika Kobayashi, Hironori Kuga, and Takuro Shimbohave pointed out that some dimension(s) of religiosity was associated with decreased fractures.[26] This research, carried out in Tokyo, is a significant fracture study due to its a large number of participants (65,898) and long data collection period of 13 years.[26] Of the 65,898 participants, the mean age was 46.2 (Standard

Deviation [SD]:12.2) years, with a 50% male-to-female ratio. During a median follow-up of 2,500 days (interquartile range (IQR):987–3,970), about 2,753(4.2%) experienced fractures, and their mean delta T-score was –0.03% (SD:18.3).[26] In multivariable longitudinal analyses, the slightly religious group had a statistically lower adjusted-odds ratio for fractures than the nonreligious group (AOR: 0.81.95% confidence interval: 0.71–0.92).[26] Hence, this piece of research concluded that 'slightly religious' participants (not 'somewhat' or 'very' religious) showed a lower incidence of fracture than non-religious individuals, although the T-scores were similar regardless of the degree of religiosity.[26] The four self-reported degrees of religiosity patients could choose included: 'not at all', or 'slightly', or 'somewhat', or 'very'. We find this study thought-provoking, as in many parts of Africa, healers state that God shows them the medicines they should use in treating patients. It was also the case that physiological and mental illnesses were attributed to the powers of ancestors or God. Thus, it is common to hear Tamnjong and other healers in this research explain that God gave them their practice and their medicines.

Traditional Healers of Ntumbaw and Njirong Villages

Pa Yerima Yongka was said to possess an enormous, in-depth knowledge of local pharmacopeia in the Western Grassfields of Cameroon. The son of Pa Yerima, David Tumi, (who had studied under his father) also went on to became a major traditional healer and set up his practice in Douala, an economic hub of the country. A fourth very famous healer in the area was known as Pa Yerimah Shokop. He lived carried out his medical practice at Shokop Quarter in Mbawrong which is in Njirong Village. His practice was also widely known and respected even beyond the northwest region, and it is claimed that some of his patients came from adjacent villages in the Western Province of Cameroon. His most well-known patient was Mr. Karngong, an educator from the Donga Mantung, who was reportedly poisoned in one of the urban towns of Cameroon. He received his initial successful detoxification, but there was a lot of internal damage, so Karngong remained ill. When he did not improve, he was brought back to the village and taken to Shokup in Mbawrong in Njirong Village, where Pa Yerima Shokop operated a traditional treatment and healing center. Karngong lived there for nearly two years. His successful treatment allowed him to return to teaching, and later, a vibrant municipality career. He was (to many residents), a testament to the efficacy of traditional medicine. The healer who treated him was not directly affiliated with any religion, but he also claimed that God had given him the knowledge to save the poisoned educator.

Social Diagnoses

In 2024, James R. Cochrane, Gary R. Gunderson, and Teresa Cutts offered their edited "Handbook on Religion and Health: Pathways for a Turbulent Future" that focused more on the intersections of communal, public, population, and planetary health, rather than on the clinical impact of religion on an individual's health.[27] Cochrane and his co-editors reordered the scholarship at the micro-, macro-, and meso-levels—analyzing broad, holistic concepts of religion and health through ecological, de-colonial, and sociological perspectives.[27] The authors point out how the Sotho language of Lesotho in southern Africa simply does not have a word for "health" that did not include all the dimensions of religion—and conversely, there is no word for "religion" that did not include all the dimensions of "health."[27] This statement demonstrates that many traditional healing practices in many parts of Africa today involve a 'meta-approach' that involves the physical, as well as the emotional, social, and spiritual dimensions of a patient. In our earlier 2017 book written by Richter, Flowers, and Bongmba entitled: "Witchcraft as a Social Diagnosis: Traditional Ghanaian Beliefs and Global Health", we learned of the foundational role that religion played in the adjudication of witchcraft accusations, as the resident healer 'diagnosed' witchcraft accusations and offered safe asylum for persons driven away for alleged witchcraft practices.[28]

Medical Ethnocentrism

Unfortunately, if we survey the literature on ethnomedicine, we can oftentimes discover the Eurocentric scholarship of 'medical ethnocentrism' in an engorged form—stuffed with proofs that native African health beliefs are sentimental and backward (or worse, childish), and sorely lacking Western biomedical treatment compliance. There are a paltry number of African medical professionals mentioned in major contemporary accounts of the history of medicine (even when the accounts are based *in* Africa and *on* Africa's tropical diseases), they infrequently add input by native medical workers.[6] Perhaps one of the most flagrant cases of 'unsung African medical heroes' was a black South African man named Hamilton Naki, who was directly involved in the first human-to-human heart transplant by Dr. Christian Barnard in December of 1967; Naki received zero credit for his efforts. Ostensibly, others include the likes of: Dr. Jean-Jacques Muyembe (Congo), who discovered the Ebola virus in 1976; African-American Dr. Charles Richard Drew (1904–1950) became the undisputed "father of blood banking" by pioneering blood preservation techniques and transfusions; Dr. Christian Happi, from Cameroon, is a molecular biologist who helped sequence the Ebola virus genome in 2014, which led to rapid diagnostic testing; and many, many more.[29] The historical heritage of medicine should never seek to silence the effect, agency, and influence of Africans who have successfully shaped, and continue to shape, compelling and robust scientific work tackling acute global challenges.

Nonetheless, there are some African medical pioneers that are currently making global headlines, like Ghanaian orthopedic surgeon Oheneba Boachie Adjei, an international authority on complex spinal surgeries, such as spinal reconstruction, kyphosis (excessive convex curvature of the spine in the thoracic and sacral regions), lordosis (abnormal inward concave lordotic curving of the cervical and lumbar regions), and scoliosis (a sideways curvature of the spine).[29] Trained in U.S., Kumas-based Boachie founded the Foundation of Orthopedics and Complex Spine (FOCOS), and FOCOS Orthopedic Hospital in Accra. According to CNN, Boachie went back to Ghana to serve his people as he said: "I don't want to be like the only person who can do this. I'd rather have four or five people who can do this. I'd rather say 'we' can do this, not just 'me.' I like 'we' better than 'I'."[29p2]

Therefore, we will continue to celebrate the achievements of these African medicine and public health pioneers that prove that determination, ambition, keen intellect, and excellence transforms global health agendas and systems. We must also work to create opportunities for future generations to follow in their footsteps, ensuring that the legacy of African researchers and physicians in medicine, orthopedic surgery, emergency medicine, etc., endures for years to come.

Five Principal Points

Firstly, recent scholarship has engaged the studies of healthcare and health systems in Africa through the lens of indigenous knowledge, which for historical reasons has been investigated through what Njoki Wane has described as an 'anti-colonial theoretical framework'.[30] Wane highlights postcoloniality as a praxis that rethinks and rejects colonial theoretical practices that undermine and reject African epistemological tools and African knowledge construction.[30] Wane appeals to African knowledge systems that have been constructed to demonstrate multiple ways of knowing (which she argues Kenyan healing practices is unveiling in different ways). Wane was part of a study of African indigenous knowledge where scholars reported that young children were knowledgeable of various herbs that were purported to have medicinal benefits.[30]

Secondly, our book is an attempt to provide a snapshot and invite further studies of traditional medicine in order to understand the local (traditional) science behind it. Here there are a number of questions which we can only raise, but not deliver tangible or definitive answers. Now given what we know about traditional medicine and healing in Africa, why is the integration of such healing systems taking such a protracted amount of time to accomplish? Also, since many of the healers attribute their practice to their ancestors (a category now recognized by scholars), what can be done to get Christian religious communities to engage in pro-active and constructive dialogue with traditional healers? Unfortunately, only the future will answer these queries.

Thirdly, our book should also be seen as a small voice added to the major declaration of traditional African medical practices; whereby each individual's experiences and contributions is shaped by their medical decisions and available wellness resources. We do not seek to undermine any advances in modern medicine, however there should be a recognition that, despite Western facilities, traditional healing continues to flourish.

Fourth, if traditional healing faces any monumental challenge today, that challenge does not come from biomedical practices, the threat comes from the common enemy of climate change. This global threat has escalated desertification to an incalculable speed—shocking farmers, agricultural workers, and other African "Guardians of the Land" (per Schoffeleers)[269] who utilize the continent's flora and fauna. (For more detailed information on deforestation, see Chapter 9, recommendation #14.)

Fifth, we want to conclude these introductory remarks by clarifying that by "emphasizing religion as a key component of traditional healing" we are not re-fetishizing medical practice in Africa. We highlight two points: first, we recognize how far traditional African healing studies has evolved (whereas early studies emphasized the symbols and medicine used by healers as fetishism); secondly, we acknowledge the shift from discourses of fetishism to traditional healers, their work, and the materials they employ.

In closing, as we end this introductory chapter, we recognize that there are, conceivably, numerous other questions we could have addressed in this book (if given unrestricted time, space, and liberty). First, can we honestly inquire how safe and efficacious traditional treatment of bone fractures is in the twenty-first century, given the advances in biosciences and medicine? An answer to this question will take us outside of the scope of this book, and unquestionably hyper-expand the scope of our inquiry. Second, many queries could be raised on the medications traditional bonesetters utilize. Could they develop these medicines on an industrial scale and get patents for these products? Regrettably, we can only attest to healer's DIY labeling and packaging of their homegrown remedies, then selling them at markets, shops, and/or along roadsides. Conceivably, many rural-area healers (who continue to unsuccessfully treat acute fractures) will continue to operate (unregulated) out of their private homes. A third question to ponder has to do with the relationship between healers, national state authorities, and their departments/ministries of health. We believe that concerning this query a successful *détente* and recognition of the role traditional healers play in public health care has been recognized for some time now. We believe that the healers and the state share a mutual interest in establishing a feasible, dynamic, and pragmatic relationship that focuses on the safe production of medicines. To wit, will the dialogue on the efficacy of the medications remain solely under the purview of each individual healer? What control can the state exercise over the healer's actions, apparatus, and production of medicines utilized by traditional bonesetters? Additionally, since many of the healers are members of their respective communities, could African states, in addition to monitoring treatment, characterize their practice as a suitable component within the confines of primary care? One could argue that this is a redundant question since many governments have recognized the efficacy of traditional or herbal healing mechanisms. However, the counter argument here is: What is in a name? If traditional bone-fracture treatment and bone-setting is effective (to such an extent that patients do not require tertiary care), what hinders these medical interventions from participating in primary healthcare systems? Fourth, would research universities expand their investigations to include the safe and regulated production of these medicines? And if they do, who would glean the recognition? The academics? Or the traditional healers who have acquired the knowledge from sheer rugged experimentation and painstaking field experience? What about the scientists who step in and provide the much-needed expertise in order to meet rigorous medical, academic, and global World Health Organization standardization? In our opinion, universities would seem to be the keen choice, as they undertake research in agriculture, urban development, ethno-medicine, and desertification. Fifth, we admit there are dire concerns and consequential disputes in the field of traditional medicine, and researchers are raising significant contentions concerning adequate R&D and the efficacious production of indigenous medicines. Online discussions attest to the fact that traditional medical practices (in which in our study has focused on bone-setting) have advanced over time, but these broad swaths of uncertainty remain—even if studies like ours celebrate what has been accomplished over the long *durée.* Some of these sociobiological concerns, including determinants of patronage, prohibitive healthcare costs, provider mistrust, and others, will be addressed in the next chapter entitled "Pathologies of Social Mechanisms".

Chapter 2

PATHOLOGIES OF SOCIAL MECHANISMS

Incongruously, LMICs in Africa account 93% of the world's fatalities on the roads (even though these countries only constitute 60% of the world's vehicles), a disproportionate sum due to conflicts and substandard emergency medical services—both which continually increase trauma burdens, according to the WHO.[31] The paradox of this Global Burden of Injury is pronounced—the poor population and active young adult age group are disproportionately affected by trauma and injury—specifically those groups requiring the best care for an improved outcome, thereby reducing the economic burden of work-time losses and life expectancies due to debilitating post-traumatic morbidities and mortalities. It can be said that the Public Health priorities of many African governmental health ministries are still focused on communicable diseases (and perhaps most recently noncommunicable diseases such as diabetes and heart disease), with trauma as the still 'forgotten stepchild of the health care system'—despite ranking as the sixth global cause of death and fifth cause of moderate and severe disabilities, according to WHO estimates.[32]

In the WHO's report: "From Burden to 'Best Buys': Reducing the Economic Impact of Non-Communicable Diseases in Low- and Middle-Income Countries," the organization stated that "83% of the 4.6 million global deaths" occur in developing countries; LMIC deaths from injuries outnumber TB, malaria and HIV diseases combined. It has been estimated if all-cause injury mortality in LMICs was reduced to the level seen in high-income countries, more than two million lives, 50 million Daily Adjusted Life Years (DALYs), and US$786 billion could be saved each year.[33]

The 'Forgotten' Pandemic of Trauma

In Rossiter's 2021 article entitled: "Trauma—The forgotten pandemic?", the author states that global mortalities, at over 6,000,000 annually from trauma, outnumber "any other single cause in the global working population" and "more than all contagious diseases added together including

COVID-19"—with the number of people injured exceeding that of any other medical condition.[34] Rossiter concurs with most research, reporting that this "Human Rights Issue" affects LMICs disproportionately at 80%–90%, with the "forgotten pandemic" of trauma presently receiving "less than 1% of global healthcare funding."[p3]

It remains an almost "incomprehensible' aberration as to why EMS (globally) continues to receive comparatively dismal funding—despite its irrefutable (and well-documented) role in the decrease or prevention of disability, higher cost of care, and fatalities. Timely and skillful EMS interventions can alleviate disabilities, deaths, speed recovery, and save money (high acuity = high costs) via proper injury prevention, skillful on-site prehospital EMS, and timely access to (a patient's matching trauma acuity 1–4 level) care system. As EMS providers, we have long-held the critical importance of a trauma patient's 'Golden Hour'—an indispensable 60-minute window where (minor) medical interventions deliver (major) survival and recovery outcomes. During this hour, appropriate prehospital care can control external hemorrhaging, ensure adequacy of ventilation (SPO2), retain patency of airway, immobilize spine (c-spine), resuscitate, and prevent environmental exposure, etc. International injury advocates must "make the case" that an improvement in trauma care translates into better population healthcare, and that the case "needs to repeatedly be made that such activity is an investment, not a cost," according to 2018s The Economist's Unit.[35p41] The gaps in orthopedic trauma (and emergency trauma care in general) require a timely intervention before it breaks existing, already limited, LMIC resources.

The warped contradiction in injuries is pronounced, as the poor and (more active) young populations are disproportionately affected by trauma and injury, and also require the best care for an improved outcome—thereby reducing loss of work time as well as the economic burden of a young population (with a long(er) life expectancy) struggling with debilitating post-traumatic morbidities. So, while governmental health ministry's still prioritize communicable diseases; trauma remains the 'unfavored underdog', even though many sub-Saharan countries are desperately burdened by horrific war injuries, road traffic fatalities, and interpersonal violence.

If we delve into our four studied African nations, we see that according to the WHO, road injuries were the top cause of mortalities in 2019 for Cameroon, Ethiopia, and Ghana, among 20- to 24-year-old males (second in Zimbabwe). See Chart 1 for details on WHO's Cause of Death by Road Injury from 2019 in DALYS (per 100,000 pop), as follows: Cameroon (all ages: 1,971.23; male and female aged 20–24 years: 2,129.58; males between 20 and 24 years old: 3,681.69); Ethiopia (all ages: 1,523.93; male and female aged 20–24 years: 1,209.63; males between 20 and 24 years old: 1,974.96);

Ghana (all ages: 1,681.43; male and female aged 20–24 years: 2,167.22; males between 20 and 24 years old: 3,575.83); and Zimbabwe (all ages: 2,166.55; male and female aged 20–24 years: 1,932.65; males between 20 and 24 years old: 3,614.12).[36] Across all four countries, we see a significant gender-disaggregated increases in the ratios of male to female deaths, especially in this "high risk" division of young male drivers. Research continues to show that, globally, young adult males are more likely to be involved in RTAs than females; almost three quarters (73%) of all road traffic deaths occur among young males (under the age of 25 years), who are almost 3 times as likely to be killed in RTAs when compared to females.[36] It would behoove public health scientists and researchers to positively exploit this sex difference in risk appetites between men and women—with programs appealing directly to the more risk-averse female population and the more risk-inclined male population.

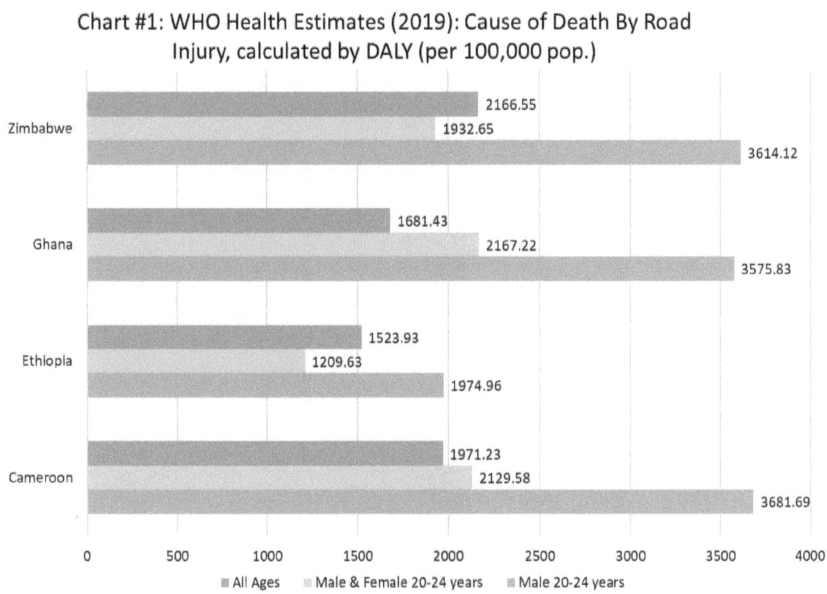

Chart 1. Cause of Death by Road Injury. Data Source: WHO, 2019.

Most organizations, including the WHO and the AO Alliance, calculate the Global Burden of Injury by using DALY, or a daily-adjusted life-year calculation. DALY is represented by the equation DALY = YLL + YLD. YLL is calculated as the number of deaths (*n*) × the standard life expectancy at age of death (L1). This measures the reduction in life expectancy. YLD is determined by the number of years disabled (weighted by level of disability caused by disease or injury) using the formula: YLD = $I \times \text{DW} \times L$ where N = number of deaths due to condition, L = standard life expectancy at age of death. Life expectancies are not the same at different ages. See Chart 1 for more information on DALY calculation. Using DALYs, we can more easily quantify the burden of diseases that cause premature death (but with no, low, or short-term disabilities, like drowning) can be compared to that of diseases that do not cause death (but do cause, for example, long-term disability (like blindness) within a specific population.

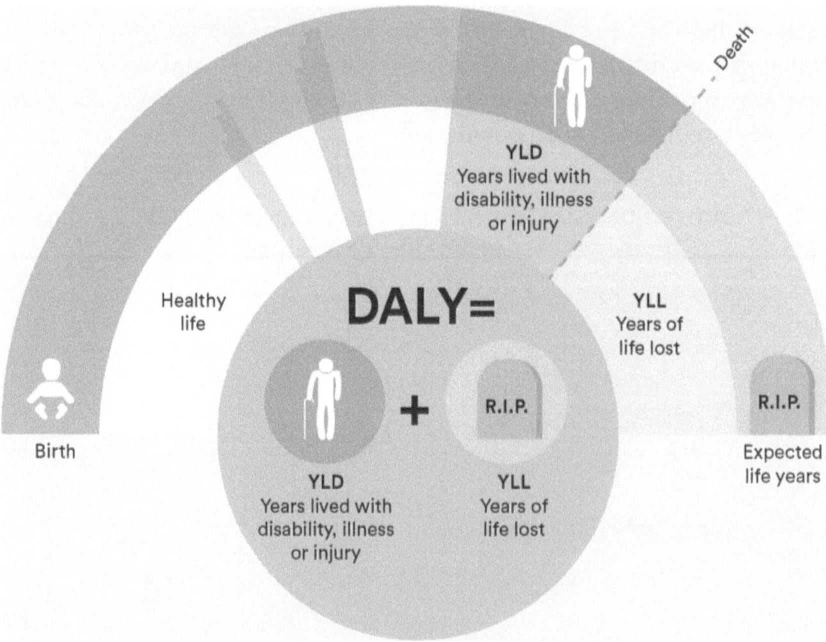

Chart 2. DALY = Disability Adjusted Life Years. Source: Public Health England, 2015.

According to the Global Burden of Disease Fracture Collaborators, a 2021 study (funded by the Bill and Melinda Gates Foundation) reported that fracture incidents were on the rise globally, with YLDs showing a precipitous increase between 1990 and 2019: Incidence increase (178 million in 2019) showed a tremendous 33.4% uptick (43.4% for women; 26.8% for men); and YLD shot up 65.3% for both men and women (71.3% for women; 60.8% for men).[37] According to the same aforementioned research study, older adults, especially women over the age of 64, were the most likely group to have new fractures; by contrast, age-specific incidence rates were 50% higher in males than in females for patients between the ages of 20 and 24.[37] Of interest were the top three anatomical fracture sites (for all ages and groups) reported by the GBD Fracture Collaborators: 1) patella, tibia or fibula, or ankle; 2) radius or ulna or both; and 3) clavicle, scapula, or humerus—with falls causing the preponderance of fractures globally.[37]

Collective Public Costs

As one example, a 2018 study performed at Makere University in Kampala, Uganda, showed that if a worker in a low-income country sustains a simple closed tibial fracture, it could take three times longer for him/her to get back to work (up to 18 months) when compared to the time it takes for a breadwinner living in a high-income country.[38] The same study in Uganda reported that within six months, the worker's children dropped out of school in order to work; regrettably, within 12 months of all of his dependents were financially struggling.[38]

Of the many studies that addressed depression and physical pain, we found the work of Sevani Singaram and Mergan Naidoo informative and instructive. Their study[38] queried 821 fracture patients, asking them to 'score' their depression (within the range 0–23); the majority (37.64%) reported 'mild depression' scores between 5 and 9 (mean of 8.26 and standard deviation of 4.76). We thought that in addition to the scientific discussion, one of the most interesting parts of Singaram and Naidoo's study was the thoughtful analysis of the psychological, financial, and occupational burdens surrounding broken bones. For example, the aforementioned study revealed that for tibial fractures (29%), healing demanded 6–20 months of recovery.[39] In general terms, white-collar workers returned to work sooner, and almost half (some 42%) used friends and family as a source of financial aid.[39] According to Singaram and Naidoo's study[39]:

> The burden of long-bone fractures impacts society through the loss of productivity, the direct and indirect costs of treatment and the additional contribution to morbidity and mortality. The management and treatment of long bone fractures add significantly to the expenses of any health care system because of the cost of surgery, possible rehospitalization and the physical rehabilitation of patients.[p1207]

We have limited the discussion of the (rather interminable) postfracture challenges to note that bone fractures not only pose problems for the individual and their families, but oftentimes ensnares elements within the patient's extended community, region, and nation. Losses of income, the shifting of resources, and the prevalence of catastrophic injuries, all serve to create huge financial burdens to individuals and their families, as well as local, regional, and national economies.

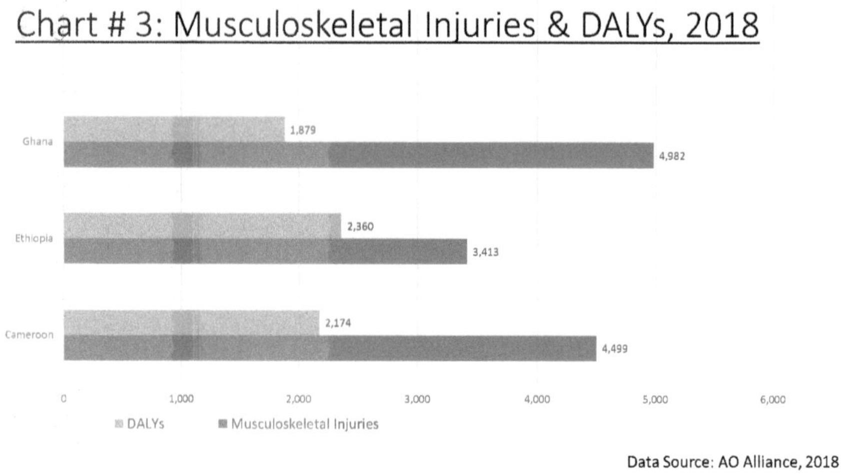

Chart 3. Cameroon, Ethiopia, and Ghana Musculoskeletal Injuries and DALYs. Zimbabwean data unavailable. Data Source: The Economist Unit, a 2018 report by AO Alliance.[35]

From Chart 3, we can see how many musculoskeletal injuries Cameroon (4,499), Ethiopia (3,413), and Ghana (4,982) suffered in 2018 alone.[35] From the same study, we see that the three nation's DALYs for Cameroon were calculated to be around 2,174, Ethiopia at 2,360, and finally, Ghana at 1,879.[35] Again, DALYs help us to calculate the economic burden that injuries and deaths have on a country's economy. Why? Because to simply state a number of mortalities does not give us a comprehensive view of individuals at different life stages, different disabilities, genders, and populations. So, the DALY is an extremely useful time-based measure that adds (YLLs—years of life not in full health) and (YLDs—years of life lost due to disability). Therefore, in Chart 3, we see that Ethiopia has the highest losses of their population's possible 'full health' when compared to Cameroon and Ghana in 2018.

In Chart 4, we see a detailed look at (only) three of the four studied nations—Cameroon, Ethiopia, and Ghana. Unfortunately, comparable data from Zimbabwe was unavailable. When we look at the aforementioned Chart 3, we can compare the cumulative losses of injury mortalities from 2015 to 2020 for Cameroon at 31.6 (per 100,000); compared to Ethiopia at 34.2 and Ghana at much higher rate of 50.4.[35] The cumulative loss to the countries in billions of U.S. Dollars (USD) is calculated at $8.67 billion for Cameroon, a staggering

$25.81 billion loss for Ethiopia, and Ghana at $6.84 billion shortfall.[35] The welfare loss (a.k.a 'deadweight loss' calculates deficits due to imbalances in production and consumption) in billions of USD was set at $3.11 billion for Cameroon, $5.58 billion for Ethiopia, and $3.15 billion for Ghana.[35] Finally, the percentage of citizens who are deemed as 'high risk' for catastrophic medical costs (which is calculated at any costs exceeding a 10% income loss) was a whopping 85% for Ethiopian citizens, 64% of Cameroonians, and conversely, only 36% for Ghanaians.[35]

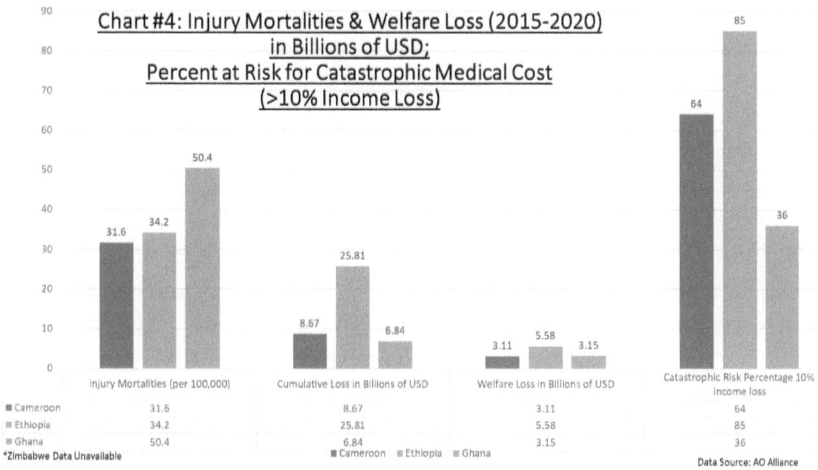

Chart 4. Shows the breakout of Injury Mortalities in billions of U.S. dollars, and the percentage of each population at risk for catastrophic costs (>10% of income). Data Source: AO Alliance.

In 2023, Ghana's National Road Safety Commission (NRSC) reported 1,600 people die (about four people per day) on its national roadways, accounting for national fiscal losses over 230 million USD annually.[40] This loss correlated to almost two percent (1.7%) of Ghana's Gross Domestic Product, with far-reaching detrimental national development effects, according to the Ghana News Agency.[40]

Pushing Back On (Any) Harmful Practices

Conventional practitioners' arguments are that TBS is riddled in 'pseudo-sciences' and inexact dosages, poor diagnoses, charlatanism, conflicts of interest, exaggerated claims of abilities, and inadequate knowledge of anatomy, lack of diagnostics (X-rays), poor hygiene, and disease transmission—all creating mistrust between the practitioners of traditional healing and modern medicine.[4] Sofowora et al.[41] and Richter et al.[42] concur with Hillenbrand[4] and have also attributed resistance to the integration of traditional medicine by the conventional medicine practitioners to primary philosophical distinctions. Conventional medicine is based on the results of experiments and views about illnesses as the result of how the pathological agents respond to various treatments; conversely, traditional medicine allows that disease can have supernatural causes. Many Western-trained physicians deem traditional or alternative healers to be charlatans, preying on the superstitions of (less-educated) communities. Just as with any field of practice this may be true in some—but not all—cases. That being said, we simply cannot deny that some TBS methods are devoid of evidence-based interventions or scientific precision (infection control, radiographic imaging, etc.) and that their (oftentimes gross) misunderstandings of human healing/physiology/anatomy have, in fact, many times over led to unnecessary complications, misalignments, improper healing, short- and long-term disabilities, infections, decreased range of motion at joints, amputations, deaths, etc.

Harmful cultural practices—like child marriage, female genital mutilation (FGM) (and we would argue any untrained, unhygienic, and unsafe bone-setting methods) are considered by UNICEF[43] to be "discriminatory practices committed regularly over such long periods of time that societies begin to consider them acceptable."[p1] From a social (peer-pressure) and cultural standpoint, bone-setting practices share some analogous orthodox roots to other entrenched sub-Saharan African rituals. FGM is defined as any procedure(s) that involves injury and/or partial (or total) removal of the external female genitalia for nonmedical reasons, according to the WHO.[44] FGM has no health benefits for girls and women, reports the WHO, and causes any number of severely debilitating injuries and lifelong illnesses, including: urination problems, painful sexual intercourse, repeated infections (which can lead to infertility), severe bleeding, cysts/abscesses, incontinence, as well as complications in childbirth and increased risk of newborn deaths.[44] Determinants of "nonvoluntary" FGM patronage, according to the BBC, include social acceptance, religion, erroneous hygiene knowledge, preservation of virginity, and enhancing male sexual pleasure.[45] Like FGM's community-led practices, bone-setting presents a considerable challenge, highlighting the need for increased prevention efforts to safeguard a growing population at risk. If we review successful strategies that have helped eradicate harmful social practices (like FGM) in the Public Health sector, we find that a broad range of "documented programmatic, research, and policy interventions," according to Williams-Breault, which are "led by a variety of national and international nongovernmental organizations and UN agencies" can encourage "communities, families, and individuals" to accept advocacy and education interventions "aimed at communities and leaders, legislative interventions, capacity-building interventions, health care interventions, media interventions, and community dialogue."[46p223] Accordingly, like FGM, it is important that there is no cultural "romanticizing"[3,47] of traditional healing practices that disfigure, maim, and cause irreparable disabilities. The debate over whether or not ethnobiology 'romanticizes' traditional practices, may, in fact, serve to impede the urgent need for more experimental clinical trial studies that can evaluate local experiences via unbiased biochemical hypothesis-testing analyses. These evidence-based findings should then be documented, publicly published via academia, safeguarded by patent, and culturally preserved (in country/*in situ*). Still, it is essential that professionals working in ethnobotanics do not don rose-colored glasses, circumvent (or spiritually/culturally bypass) hard scientific discovery, and lean into public sentiment of exploitive familial- or community-based loyalties.

Truthfully, in retrospect, if we look back over the ages at the historical pathways of how traditional midwifery practices evolved, they too began as a 'harmful' community-led medical practice; only to (now) become a reasonably standardized, organized, integrated, and professionally registered praxis over many decades in many countries [...] So then, why not traditional bone-setting procedures? For they too, began as no more than communal spheres of collected successful and unsuccessful treatment experiences, moving step by step into a globally accepted practice of primary (low risk, rudimentary, nonsurgical) medical care. In truth, the systemic impact of trained Traditional Birth Attendants (TBAs) to alleviate burgeoning obstetrical patient numbers, hospital/clinic overcrowding, as well as the continuity of wellness care by a midwife for both mother and child—cannot be underestimated. And therein remains the positive expectancies of allowing the integration of TBS into the orthodox fold. Certainly, it bears a working trial should both segments embrace the changes to their roles and reputations.

First Rule: Do No Harm

While the veracity of documented medical claims against some traditional bonesetter methods cannot be denied (as they are physical records of radiological, clinical, and physiological evidence)—the cultural ethno-ethics involved in TBS is much more convoluted, mired in supernatural philosophies, intimate personal and familial relationships, as well as shared community identity. We found that Ewuoso et al.,[48] a medical ethics professor, was one of the few African researchers who boldly published TBS's "rendezvous in quackery" and inherent bioethical immorality of traditional bonesetters who "cross the line" by purposefully delaying limb/life-threatening physician referrals and using "pseudo-scientific practices with little (or no) benefits to patients."[p2] Ewuoso added that the fact that "nearly all" TBS are "unlicensed and unqualified" to render care makes their diagnostic (or lack thereof) and treatment methods "no longer ethically defensible."[p6] With that, it is perplexing to observe the African communities' rather tacit sanctioning of TBS' (obvious) conflict of interest—whereby bonesetter's judgment concerning patient welfare is improperly influenced by underlying (secretive) interest(s) such as financial gain or public recognition. Therefore, some medical studies have recommended a complete elimination (or gradual phasing out) of TBS care, while others, concede that there is an inherent futility in uprooting such an entrenched art patronized by all levels of African society.

Long considered to be the First Rule of Medicine for every Western-trained physician, nurse, paramedic, or therapist—the principle of 'DO NO HARM' gives every patient the right not to be harmed and to have the risk of harm minimized while receiving health-based care. Within this "first, do no harm" (in its original Latin: *primum non nocere*) principle of medical ethics, patients' rights include the full disclosure of the likelihood of benefit, known risks and side effects of the proposed treatment, any viable alternative treatments, as well as the entire exposure range of unknown risks—all to benefit the patient in assessing the risk-to-reward ratio in their consent to the specified provider's treatment plan. Therefore, every healthcare provider pledges to abstain from all intentional wrong-doing and purposeful harm during their ministrations, counsel, and conduct.

As Ewuoso et al. stated in their published *Journal of Public Health Reports* 2021 article: "Ubuntu Ethics and Moral Problems in Traditional Bone-Healing"[48]:

> The greatest threat to the ethical reflection on TBH which we provide in this study might be the argument that TBH is a traditional care practice, and the people love their traditional heritage. It would, thus, be difficult to ask individuals to abandon their heritage. Some also pointed that traditional bone services are too prevalent, and the patronage is too high to be easily replaced by modern medicine [...] this study argues that prevalence is not a sufficient reason for incorporating TBH services in the healthcare system or claiming that they are indispensable. Moreover, in a study conducted by Onyemaechi and colleagues, about 90% of study participants think that traditional bone services are dispensable in their communities. An argument derived from prevalence, for incorporating TBH services in the healthcare system, can easily lead to ethical drift [...] Ubuntu ethic emphasizes relational values of communion, as well

> as incorporates other important values like beneficence, relational autonomy, and a commitment to avoidable harm. **A commitment to avoidable harm** might imply, in this context, the need to revise or avoid the diagnostic and treatment methods that have been shown by empirical data, to complicate patient care.[p8]

From a legal standpoint, none of the TBS studied had obtained any legal practice permit under the auspices of their national Ministry of Health (despite practicing for many years). Without any legal authority or licensing overseeing TBS's operations, it is nearly impossible for government entities to identify, control, and/or enforce a 'standard' for the quality in bonesetter services; furthermore, bonesetter patients cannot be afforded any legal protection in case of negligence, malpractice, or misconduct by bonesetters. With few exceptions, there are no well-known published global cases that attest to traditional bonesetter malpractice suits in courts of national law. There was an interesting lawsuit in the United States from December 17, 1883, between James Warren and his bonesetter "Dr. Sweet" in Connecticut, as reported in "Suing a Natural Bonesetter; a Connecticut Dr. Sweet and the Family He Sprang From," as reported by the *New York Times*.[49]

In another case in 1976, Yeung Yuk Kee (Plaintiff) sued Kong Tsing Bor (Defendant) in the High Court of Hong Kong as she had been injured in a car accident in 1975, and underwent successful surgery of all five fingers of her right hand (Judgment # HCA2957/1975).[50] After discharge from the hospital, she consulted a bonesetter almost daily between May and December, and the bonesetter instructed her to be noncompliant with hospital's prescribed physical therapy regimen.[50] So, without any movement, the finger muscles atrophied and her hand lacked flexion. Now the question before the court was: Is the plaintiff's (apparent) permanent disability due to her own willful act? Legally speaking, in Hong Kong, a plaintiff cannot recover damages "for an aggravation or prolongation of his injuries which is due to his own willful act or neglect," and as J. Lush said in *Jones v. Watney, Combe, Reid & Co., Ltd.* (1912), 28 T.L.R. 399:

> The jury must look at all the circumstances of the case, the medical advice received, the need for action, the usual character of what is actually done, and the precautions taken during the doing of it. The injured person need not act with perfect knowledge and wisdom, but, upon the other hand, cannot claim damages for such injuries as are really due to wanton, heedless, or careless conduct on his own part (High Court of Hong Kong, *Yeung Yuk Kee v. Kong Tsing Bor*, July 20, 1976).[50pl]

Malpractice: Failure To Act Is an Act

Today, a complication like nonunion is seen (globally) as representing a poor standard of care, and the malpractice cases reflect both a 'defensive litigious medical culture' and a zero-tolerance stance for (avoidable) Western medical errors. To put it succinctly, failure to act—is an act. When bonesetters fail to recognize that the disease process or injury is beyond their ability to assess or manage—it is incumbent upon them to acknowledge that they are unable to adequately care for the patient. So, when a patient presents to a traditional bonesetter with a soft-tissue mass (a possible tumor) on their leg or arm, they should immediately refer the patient to a higher level of medical care. In Western healthcare professions, purposeful delays of referring the patient to a higher standard of care is considered malpractice. Malpractice usually involves a patient making a legal claim for compensation claiming that their healthcare provider and/or hospital facility allowed medical error(s) in the proper diagnosis, medication dosage, and/or treatment that adversely impacted the patient's prognosis. However, in order to claim malpractice, a patient must prove that their care fell short of established standards and caused him/her harm. In fact, there are four specific criteria that must be met so as to bring about a successful legal medical malpractice suit in the United States, and they are sometimes referred to as the four "D's." The four "D's" of medical malpractice are Duty, Dereliction (or Deviation), Damages, and Direct Cause—all four must be proven in a court in law in order to claim negligence and be awarded any restitution.[51] According to Epker's article published in Forbes magazine: 1) Duty of care (care that is proven to be "below the standard expected of a similarly trained and reasonably competent professional"); 2) Dereliction of duty (purposeful negligence); 3) Damages (like suffering, constant pain, considerable loss of income, or disability); as well as 4) Direct cause.[51]

In Epker's 2024 article: "Truly Unsustainable: The Effect of Medical Malpractice on Caregiving," the Forbes magazine journalist explains that U.S. doctors, paramedics, and nurses are practicing 'defensive CYA medicine' in such "a litigious environment, it creates a sense of fear," and these emerging 'nuclear verdicts' (>$10 million) emit a chilling effect on accessibility, cost, and quality of care for all Americans.[51] There are an unlimited number of side-effects by healthcare practitioners due to this extreme environ, including, but not limited to: less 'open' doctor–patient communication, overdocumentation via notes and patient charting, increased second opinion consults, and perhaps the costliest effect of all—unnecessary scans, test, and procedures that are ordered in the hopes of alleviating the onus of possible future malpractice claims.[51]

Ethically Speaking

Most assuredly, one of the earliest oaths of medical ethics was written by the Greek physician Hippocrates (460–370 BC) sometime between the fifth and third centuries BC. The updated secular 1960s version (see below) of the oath is publicly sworn, to this very day, by new physicians at medical universities throughout the Western world. Very much like the African concept of Ubuntu, the Hippocratic oath explicitly outlines ethical measures such as gratitude, compassion, justice, honesty, humbleness, sanctity, integrity, confidentiality, fidelity to the bond, non-malfeasance (an illegal or immoral act that causes the patient physical or monetary harm), and respect for human life and dignity.

The Hippocratic Oath, in Greek (1923 Loeb edition), and the English translation[52]:

ὄμνυμι Ἀπόλλωνα ἰητρὸν καὶ Ἀσκληπιὸν καὶ Ὑγείαν καὶ Πανάκειαν καὶ θεοὺς πάντας τε καὶ πάσας, ἵστορας ποιεύμενος, ἐπιτελέα ποιήσειν κατὰ δύναμιν καὶ κρίσιν ἐμὴν ὅρκον τόνδε καὶ συγγραφὴν τήνδε:

I swear by Apollo Healer, by Asclepius, by Hygieia, by Panacea, and by all the gods and goddesses, making them my witnesses, that I will carry out, according to my ability and judgment, this oath and this indenture.

ἡγήσεσθαι μὲν τὸν διδάξαντά με τὴν τέχνην ταύτην ἴσα γενέτῃσιν ἐμοῖς, καὶ βίου κοινώσεσθαι, καὶ χρεῶν χρηΐζοντι μετάδοσιν ποιήσεσθαι, καὶ γένος τὸ ἐξ αὐτοῦ ἀδελφοῖς ἴσον ἐπικρινεῖν ἄρρεσι, καὶ διδάξειν τὴν τέχνην ταύτην, ἢν χρηΐζωσι μανθάνειν, ἄνευ μισθοῦ καὶ συγγραφῆς, παραγγελίης τε καὶ ἀκροήσιος καὶ τῆς λοίπης ἁπάσης μαθήσιος μετάδοσιν ποιήσεσθαι υἱοῖς τε ἐμοῖς καὶ τοῖς τοῦ ἐμὲ διδάξαντος, καὶ μαθητῇσι συγγεγραμμένοις τε καὶ ὡρκισμένοις νόμῳ ἰητρικῷ, ἄλλῳ δὲ οὐδενί.

To hold my teacher in this art equal to my own parents; to make him partner in my livelihood; when he is in need of money to share mine with him; to consider his family as my own brothers, and to teach them this art, if they want to learn it, without fee or indenture; to impart precept, oral instruction, and all other instruction to my own sons, the sons of my teacher, and to indentured pupils who have taken the Healer's oath, but to nobody else.

διαιτήμασί τε χρήσομαι ἐπ' ὠφελείῃ καμνόντων κατὰ δύναμιν καὶ κρίσιν ἐμήν, ἐπὶ δηλήσει δὲ καὶ ἀδικίῃ εἴρξειν.

οὐ δώσω δὲ οὐδὲ φάρμακον οὐδενὶ αἰτηθεὶς θανάσιμον, οὐδὲ ὑφηγήσομαι συμβουλίην τοιήνδε: ὁμοίως δὲ οὐδὲ γυναικὶ πεσσὸν φθόριον δώσω.

ἁγνῶς δὲ καὶ ὁσίως διατηρήσω βίον τὸν ἐμὸν καὶ τέχνην τὴν ἐμήν.

οὐ τεμέω δὲ οὐδὲ μὴν λιθιῶντας, ἐκχωρήσω δὲ ἐργάτῃσιν ἀνδράσι πρήξιος τῆσδε.

ἐς οἰκίας δὲ ὁκόσας ἂν ἐσίω, ἐσελεύσομαι ἐπ' ὠφελείῃ καμνόντων, ἐκτὸς ἐὼν πάσης ἀδικίης ἑκουσίης καὶ φθορίης, τῆς τε ἄλλης καὶ ἀφροδισίων ἔργων ἐπί τε γυναικείων σωμάτων καὶ ἀνδρῴων, ἐλευθέρων τε καὶ δούλων.

ἃ δ' ἂν ἐνθεραπείῃ ἴδω ἢ ἀκούσω, ἢ καὶ ἄνευ θεραπείης κατὰ βίον ἀνθρώπων, ἃ μὴ χρή ποτε ἐκλαλεῖσθαι ἔξω, σιγήσομαι, ἄρρητα ἡγεύμενος εἶναι τὰ τοιαῦτα.

ὅρκον μὲν οὖν μοι τόνδε ἐπιτελέα ποιέοντι, καὶ μὴ συγχέοντι, εἴη ἐπαύρασθαι καὶ βίου καὶ τέχνης δοξαζομένῳ παρὰ πᾶσιν ἀνθρώποις ἐς τὸν αἰεὶ χρόνον: παραβαίνοντι δὲ καὶ ἐπιορκέοντι, τἀναντία τούτων.

I will use those dietary regimens which will benefit my patients according to my greatest ability and judgment, and I will do no harm or injustice to them. Neither will I administer a poison to anybody when asked to do so, nor will I suggest such a course. Similarly, I will not give to a woman a pessary to cause abortion. But I will keep pure and holy both my life and my art. I will not use the knife, not even, verily, on sufferers from stone, but I will give place to such as are craftsmen therein.

Into whatsoever houses I enter, I will enter to help the sick, and I will abstain from all intentional wrongdoing and harm, especially from abusing the bodies of man or woman, bond or free. And whatsoever I shall see or hear in the course of my profession, as well as outside my profession in my intercourse with men, if it be what should not be published abroad, I will never divulge, holding such things to be holy secrets.

Now if I carry out this oath, and break it not, may I gain for ever reputation among all men for my life and for my art; but if I break it and forswear myself, may the opposite befall me.

The far more secular version (a.k.a 'modern version') was written in 1964 by Louis Lasagna, Academic Dean of the School of Medicine at Tufts University, and is still used by medical schools today[53]:

> I swear to fulfill, to the best of my ability and judgment, this covenant: I will respect the hard-won scientific gains of those physicians in whose steps I walk, and gladly share such knowledge as is mine with those who are to follow. I will apply, for the benefit of the sick, all measures [that] are required, avoiding those twin traps of overtreatment and therapeutic nihilism. I will remember that there is art to medicine as well as science, and that warmth, sympathy, and understanding may outweigh the surgeon's knife or the chemist's drug. I will not be ashamed to say 'I know not', nor will I fail to call in my colleagues when the skills of another are needed for a patient's recovery. I will respect the privacy of my patients, for their problems are not disclosed to me that the world may know. Most especially must I tread with care in matters of life and death. If it is given me to save a life, all thanks. But it may also be within my power to take a life; this awesome responsibility must be faced with great humbleness and awareness of my own frailty. Above all, I must not play at God. I will remember that I do not treat a fever chart, a cancerous growth, but a sick human being, whose illness may affect the person's family and economic stability. My responsibility includes these related problems, if I am to care adequately for the sick. I will prevent disease whenever I can, for prevention is preferable to cure. I will remember that I remain a member of society, with special obligations to all my fellow human beings, those sound of mind and body as well as the infirm. If I do not violate this oath, may I enjoy life and art, respected while I live and remembered with affection thereafter. May I always act so as to preserve the finest traditions of my calling and may I long experience the joy of healing those who seek my help.[53]

On the other side of the world, in Persia, a medical ethicist was born in 980 AD, known as Avicenna (a.k.a. the "Prince of Physicians"). A keen student of Aristotle, Avicenna treatise in five volumes of the *al-Qanun fi al-Tibb* (or The Canon of Medicine) considering: patient interests ("He should not prescribe therapeutics unaffordable for patient"); patient confidentiality ("the physician ought to protect the patient's secrets" and should not "express patient diseases such as hemorrhoids and diseases of women except in the cases of necessity and (only) to the people who should know"); communication skills (stay "away from extremes of intimacy or arrogance; because excessive intimacy and jesting harm the dignity of physician while arrogance or any harshness could harm the patient–physician relationship"[54]; and adhering to the very detailed characteristics of professional excellence:

> "The physician should also be calm and dignified in his behavior, associated with patience gentleness and tolerance; he must listen well to the patient's complaints, explain the information he needs according to the patient's understanding, and avoid using difficult words in the conversation with the patient" [...] and "upon visiting of a patient, the physician should sit next to him in a way that is in front of him so that he could see his face and listen to him well. He should only ask the questions that provide necessary information for his diagnosis and treatment: the physician ought to avoid extraneous and unnecessary questions. Moreover, the physicians should avoid prolonging the time of his visit even if the patient wants his companion. The physician should limit the visiting time to the required length in a compassionate and respectful manner." (from Avicenna's "Canon of Medicine")[54]

It is the TBS' lack of beneficial (community) and respectful (individual) care that breaks down and damages the proverbial African concept of a shared pursuit for the common good, or Ubuntu. Made famous by South African archbishop Desmond Tutu, the Zulu term of Ubuntu "*umuntu ngumuntu ngabantu*" can be translated as "A person is a person through other people," and that the communal relationship in the Ubuntu ethic is a "*prima facie*" solidarity framework which can be used to "ground"[p2] safe and effective fracture care that is unencumbered by conflicts of interests—all remaining respectful to Africa's common public health good.[48] The South Africa-based ethics professor goes on to write that the application of Ubuntu ethics to traditional bone-setting practices could enhance community engagement processes, help negotiate consent, reconcile conflicting opinions, coalesce public compliance, and reduce exploitive TBS practitioners that are recognized and identified as harmful 'quacks' within the community. The alacritous promotion of fraudulent or ignorant medical practices is never in the best interest of the patient, nor the community. We can lean into the old age-adage: 'A robber demands your money ***or*** your life; but a quack demands your money ***and*** your life'.

Familiarity and Fear: Determinants of Patronage

There have been numerous qualitative bonesetter studies that have reported any number of reasons for TBS patronage, some include: fear of casts, implants and foreign objects including musculoskeletal traction devices; belief in the spiritual powers of the bonesetter; quick service; lack of transportation (i.e.) convenience/accessibility and flexibility of nearby or at-home treatment setting; prohibitive cost of hospitalized orthopedic care; family influence or peer-pressure; mistrust/poor perception/hostile reception at hospital facility; hospital overcrowding; misleading advertising/mass media misrepresentations and interviews; and familiarity with bonesetter culture versus lack of familiarity with orthopedic centers.[55–57] For instance, Idris et al. in 2010 showed that preferences for traditional bonesetters among 199 Sudanese patients with fractures consisted of three main beliefs: at 37%, participants prefer fracture care competencies of TBS; 14.06% liked the lower cost of TBS care; 14.06% feared the usage of plaster casts, with the remaining patients reporting a lack of treatment options due to unfeasible travel distances.[56] Interestingly, Makoge et al.'s Cameroon study in 2017, showed that university students and camp dwellers viewed hospitals and clinics as "the last resort" when they were ill, preferring to self-medicate "using available tablets, herbs, or other traditional medicines," consultations with pharmacies and/or 'unofficial Quart-doctors' (pre-med students in their 'quarter' or neighborhood).[58]

The complexity of the situation was expressed by one person who told the researchers that as an adult he had the confidence to manage his own affairs, and he only resorted to buying medicine from a chemist (modern drug store) if traditional remedies did not work. Surely public health services in Cameroon, Ethiopia, Ghana, and Zimbabwe should better anticipate people's health behaviors so they can more effectively address fracture treatment challenges among local patient populations. At this point in our discussion, we will attempt to unpack some of these specified determinants of patronage.

Prohibitive Western Medical Costs

When we review fracture care costs in each country, current and definitive costs are hard to pin down. In 2018, the *Economist* magazine reported that in Yaoundé, Cameroon, approximately 8,613 CFA was required ($18.25 USD) to gain help, or about one week's salary.[35] Unfortunately, these locally unaffordable medical expenses have consequences, explained Dr. Lekina Florent Anicet, a physician at General Hospital in Yaoundé: "Many patients are too poor to afford treatment and go to traditional healers," and added that "Most cases become handicapped for life as they did not get the right treatment. It's a very serious problem."[35p18] Plus, the current formal healthcare system in Cameroon (and many other LMICs) utilize a fee-for-service model, whereby patients are forced to pay all (or most) of their surgical and hospital stay costs up front, as well as purchase the (usually itemized) list of disposable supplies (IV catheters, syringes, bandages, wound dressings, etc.) and medication (bags of IV fluid, antibiotics, etc.) from the hospital pharmacy or local drugstore.[59]

According to Akakpo (2024), insurance schemes, like the National Health Insurance Scheme in Ghana, supports patients in the hospital; however, does not "cover critical healthcare services in relation to fractures," including supplies and services like drugs, surgery, X-rays, Plaster of Paris (POP), bandages, and so on.[60p374] These well-known 'cash-and-carry' sub-Saharan African hospital systems demand that patients purchase these supplies at local pharmacies and/or deposits funds (up front) prior to treatment. The aforementioned author succinctly illustrates these expenditures through a field interview in Ho, Ghana, in his article: "Why Patients Patronize the Services of Traditional Bone Setters: A Phenomenological Analysis of Lived Experiences of Patients in Volta Region, Ghana"[60]:

> When I suffered my fracture in 2017 and went to the hospital, I spent almost Gh¢3,000.00 (approx. $512.05 USD). As part of the treatment process, the POP was applied. The first time I went for review, I paid Gh¢800.00 (approx. $136.54 USD) after the POP was removed and a new one applied. I paid other monies in relation to drugs, the X-rays and other related costs. Not everybody can afford this amount of money at the hospital. Even with all these payments, I did not get the needed relief. I had to move to a traditional bone setter at Dodome-Dogblome. When I got there, the man told me that he would charge me Gh¢500.00 (approx. $85.47USD) but I will pay this money after successful healing. I started walking after three weeks and when I was finally healed, I paid him.[p1347]

Conversely, a documented patient in Cameroon, according to Dickson et al., indicated that he had to transfer to several centers, searching for physician who would treat his fracture. Finally, he was sent to a referral hospital for X-rays, consultation, and laboratory testing, a treatment that cost 300,000 CFA Francs ($550), forcing the patient and his family to sell some of their belongings.[59]

The cash-and-carry approach of African hospitals treks in direct opposition to traditional practitioners, who normally expect payment after his/her services are rendered. "*I accept whatever they give me*" seems to be the transactional business mantra from rural-area bonesetters concerning the expected payment for their services. These services are dependent on the severity of the injury, length of healing time, and (overall) affordability to the community at large. While cost of treatment is certainly a major consideration, the people's perception of the care is also quite important. There is a very strong innate trust in their native healers that permeates the individual realities, especially in more rural pastoral areas. Even in large cities though, native healers are many times more trusted, while Western-style hospitals and physicians are perceived as foreign interlopers. These strong communal biases can be very hard to overcome.

Oftentimes when interviewed, the bonesetter's stated they would accept whatever their clients considered adequate payment for their services. For instance, three payment methods reported for TBS services in northern Tanzania, according to Card et al.,[61] included bundling costs, livestock barter, and sliding-scale pricing. To be sure, it seems as though the continued acceptance of 'bartered services' that allow patients to purchase TBS services in exchange for cloth, guinea fowl, fruits, vegetables, chickens, etc., may be an extremely significant (albeit unexplored) 'driving force' behind the reliance on TBS in more pastoral areas. This 'behind-the-scenes' entrenched and institutionalized motivation—the ability to exchange goods for services (rather than utilizing hard currency)—is upheld by various studies in Ghana, Ethiopia, Nigeria, and Tanzania.[61–63]

Some women we interviewed off the record indicated that they only access more expensive modern healthcare facilities for the sake of her children. One woman stated that she when she falls ill, she turns to herbs, or seeks medicines via a chemist. She takes her children only to the chemist (pharmacy) because she believed they would get a proper diagnosis and better (albeit more costly) treatment. She stated that the wellbeing of her children was a priority for her.

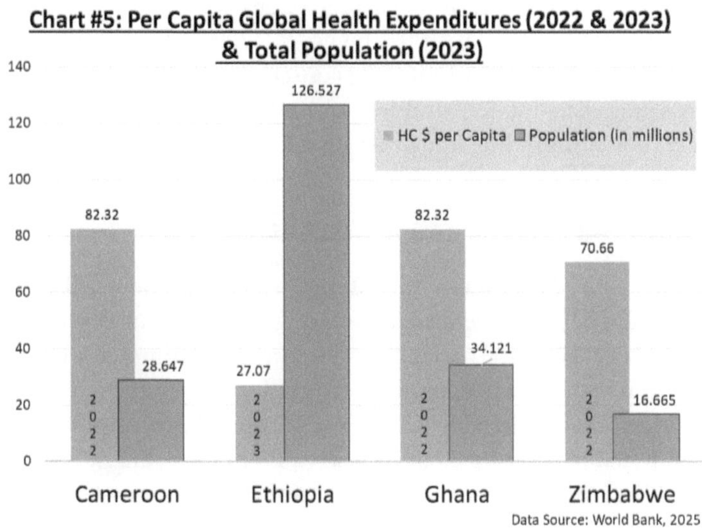

Chart 5. Per Capita WHO Global Health Expenditures. Data Source: World Bank, 2025.

When we attempt a comparative analysis of per-capita health expenditures by country, we see some distressing spending by governments, particularly in Ethiopia, where we see an almost 40% dip in comparable healthcare expenditures, despite its sizeable population. In Chart 5, we see that Cameroon spent about $72 on healthcare per capita in 2022 on their 28.64 million (2023) population; in Ethiopia, we see that approximately $27 was spent per capita in 2023 on their 126.527 million population in 2023; with Ghana, we see the highest per capita spending on healthcare at almost $82 per capita in 2022 for their 34.12 million population; and finally, we see that Zimbabwean government spent about $70 in health expenditures in 2022 for their 16.66 million population.[64] These aforementioned government expenditures consist of all expenditures "or outlays for medical care, prevention, promotion, rehabilitation, community health activities, medical education and training, and research and development, health administration and regulation and capital formation with the predominant objective of improving health" according to the Hong Kong Food and Health Bureau.[50] What is relevant to note from these macroeconomic numbers is the importance—and value—that the country has placed on their population's healthcare needs.

Contrarywise, TBS healing is not always the cheaper option in fracture care. Case in point: in Zambia wherein "despite poverty and higher costs of treatment from a traditional healer, people still frequently decide to seek treatment from a traditional healer."[65p78] Meanwhile, due to deforestation, over-harvesting, and an ever-growing scarcity of "rare" and/or endangered medicinal plants—there have been precipitous jumps in medicinal plants' costs—some as much as 50%–100% higher in Nigeria (from 2018 to 2022).[66p1] So, notwithstanding an ever-flattening cost-curve of pricing, 'real' all-natural medicines may become less and less cost-effective for the average African consumer, notwithstanding any pro-TBS efforts.

Outnumbered: Access and Availability

Cameroon, with 27 million inhabitants, reported about 40 orthopedic surgeons in 2023.[67] In some urban areas of Cameroon, the doctor-to-patient ratio is 1:150 per day in the national territory, and wait times to see a physician can be 8 hours—meanwhile, patients can find staff members that reportedly treat patients "inconsiderately," are "poorly trained and unmotivated," and unwilling to tell patients the "nature and cause of their illness."[3p286]

In 2021, in Ghana, there were only 52 trauma and orthopedic Ghanaian surgeons for a population of over 30 million.[40] If you do the math, that's an unsustainable 577,000 persons per traumatologist. Ghanaian health experts say 60% of trauma cases are road traffic accidents (RTAs), however, the majority of RTA victims elect to seek TBS care, as they unable to get the needed services from hospitals.[40]

Despite the spoken and unspoken rivalries between orthodox and unorthodox practitioners, some physicians readily acknowledge the claim of bonesetters as providers "of last resort" for millions living in rural, underserved segments of sub-Saharan African society, one Nigerian orthopedic surgeon had this to say about TBS services:

> They are filling the vacuum, because there are so many places where they don't have even a [single] doctor. They don't even have a general practitioner, not to even talk of specialist or somebody who specializes in orthopedics. In those places, if somebody has a fracture, where does the person go? There is usually somebody who attends to them. So, my perception of them is that they are filling a gap or a vacuum that has been created by lack of orthopedics. The truth is, we don't have enough orthopedists in the country. How many do we have? Only about 400-and something registered.[68p4] (participant 8, orthopedist focus group)

By and large, studies also show a pronounced difference in patient-centered approaches between traditional healers and Western-trained physicians. A Cameroon study by Labhardt et al.[69] reported significant departures in care: traditional healers diagnosed 77% of studied patients based on traditional beliefs and focused more on "psychosocial" daily life issues (10% vs. 1.4%) than on "purely medical questions," and asked for patient's opinions more—a more "psychosomatic approach" to actively seek "common ground" with their patients.[p1106] Contrariwise, Western-trained physicians in the same aforementioned study pronounced 90% of their patients with somatic (physiological) medical issues, gave information only 14.9% of the time (compared to 42.5% of TH), in 2.5% of their visit asked the patients direct questions (vs. 9.4%), and patients verbally agreed only 7.8% of the time, compared to 17.8% of the time with traditional healers.[69] Therein lies several significant issues to unpack inherent values of patient-centered approaches to care, but also the authoritarian 'godlike doctor' persona attached to uber-educated MDs by the general public. Both serve to set the stage for patient fear and/or intimidation, as well as dismissive, arrogant, and even abusive interactions with medical care providers. A 2018 study reported that 16.6% of patients had no doctor–patient relationships, so the local bonesetter in Hafizabad, Pakistan, was their preferred provider.[70] Again, there is an opportunity for empathy in that medical professionals (like any other human) can suffer 'burnout' and become overwhelmed by their demanding workloads, long hours, high-stakes (life or death) decision-making, poor patient prognosis, patient deaths (especially pediatric patients), all in addition to their everyday life stressors. So, it is important that both traditional healers and Western-trained physicians are viewed through a balanced perspective as any fellow human; having limitations, unable to perform miracles, or even guarantee perfect patient outcomes.

Supernatural Calling

While Western-trained physicians focus (almost solely) on the biomedical mechanisms and Western etiologies of illness and disease, traditional healers and bonesetters are known to take a more holistic (natural + supernatural) approach to wellbeing. Bonesetters will claim their gift of healing as an inheritance from God, oftentimes a gift they did not ask for, but rather were "called upon" to undertake via a familial legacy. In Zimbabwe, for instance, traditional healers are reputed to divine the cause of a person's illness or social problems by throwing bones to interpret the will of dead ancestors. Some healers say they directly channel the ancestral spirit through their bodies. Many have in-depth knowledge of plant materials and their various curative powers. They use leaves, seeds, stems, bark, or roots to treat symptoms. Animal parts, charms, amulets, etc., are also employed, but to a lesser extent. Most traditional healers are both herbalists and diviners, but some specialize in one aspect. Many proponents of traditional medicine claim that the long-standing history (prior to the introduction of Western medicine), close community relations, and deep cultural 'social currency' gives them precedence over Western practitioners. Case in point: a Nigerian TBS was quoted in a 2020 study[68] as saying:

> There are many severe cases that have been brought, severe cases that the hospital could not handle that in my own very eyes—we have handled them. The sweeter part of it is the testimonies we get, that a patient will come, leg or hand, or any part of the body broken. At the end of the day, within the span of three weeks, one month, the person is walking on his own without holding any staff, without anybody supporting the person. It gives you joy as a practitioner. The person comes with testimonies, with gifts; no matter how little, appreciation is appreciation.[68] (Participant 4, TBS Focus Group)

Idris et al. explained that bone-setting is popular in Africa because "its practitioners lay claim to supernatural influences," and that, "Superstition, ignorance, and poverty are the basis for continued patronage despite complications"[p199] attributed to TBS services.[56] Idris goes on to state that the high rate of return to orthodox Western care "suggests that people's confidence in the TBS is highly misplaced," and that, "their internal locus of control in decision-making is reawakened by TBS failure."[56p200] The same researcher concluded that the continued preference of TBS by Sudanese people was based on their belief that TBS are "better in treating fractures," more readily available/attainable, nearby (local or close to neighboring area), and that TBS care results in "faster healing and relief"[p204] when compared to that offered by Western biomedical options.[56] Interviews of bonesetters on mass media (TV, radio shows, etc.: media that are considered credible sources of information by rural communities) promote misleading advertisements by spiritual healers and traditional bonesetters regarding their outrageously successful practices. Sometimes, influential and popular culture personalities lend their support to TBS practices in Ethiopia (without seeking out peer-reviewed evidence-based findings).[71]

In addition to physical massage, traction (with rocks, stones), fasting, warm water compresses, bathing, dietary changes, palpation, scarification (thought to accelerate penetration of topical poultices), and/or reduction of the affected limb, some TBS depend on the invocation and summonsing of God-given spiritual, ancestral (a.k.a. powers of the bloodline; using family ties or bloodline links), and/or supernatural healing abilities. Some have reported to use divinations or incantations (during which they receive "healing powers" from their ancestors or gods).[62,72] Some bonesetters in Northern Ghana also called on superstation to ascertain a victim's expected healing period. Conversely, any TBS' inability to heal a patient's fracture can be blamed on "other forces such as the severity of the initial injury, ancestral spirits, or attacks by perceived enemies."[48p6] In the same study, the researchers claim that TBS will deliberately "withhold detailed information" about a particular patient's diagnosis/prognosis, for "fear of offending the supernatural beings"[p6] (which can, consequently, adversely affect the patient's treatment and/or outcome).[48] Yempabe et al.[62] reported that 14% of the TBS asked the patient's family to supply a chicken (mimic the patient's injury) by breaking the chicken's wing (for upper extremity fracture) or leg (lower extremity fracture) [...] direct observation of the chicken's healing injury is then undertaken—whereby the day the chicken is able to walk or use it's wing again—is considered the self-appointed day that the patient will be asked to walk or use their arm.

Conversely, patients seek 'supernatural' diagnosis and healing for their (perceived) 'supernatural' illness. Vastly differing from Western concept of disease or illness, some patients in Cameroon reported illnesses "such as '*biya*' (crossing something on your way that brings bad destiny)"; or '*kong*' (psychiatric symptoms behind your soul being sold by someone to someone else); and '*oedip*' (vaginal or urethral discharge often tied to loss of femineity).[69p1101] Any bonesetter's purposeful intent of injurious concealment, mystification, and/or fetishism of a patient's condition (based on fame, social recognition, and/or profit-based motives) should be never be tolerated by any civilized society.

Fear of Surgery, Amputation, and Casts

It has been reported that significant percentages of patients harbored (various) erroneous apprehension(s), well-earned deficient care status, and/or poor past experiences at entering Western medical facilities. Ironically, it is the exact same fear of hospital care that sends patients to traditional healers—that can, in turn, send them right back to the hospital with a profoundly delayed presentation, and (now) a permanent gait impairment, amputation, disability, etc. Subsequently when the patient presents at the hospital, despite all of its many modern equipment and techniques, some TBS patients find their (what was previously a simple remediable fracture), to have deteriorated into an acute irremediable case of osteomyelitis (bone infection), wet gangrene, or fatal sepsis. One particular bonesetter study recorded an astonishing 34% of TBS patient cases that were deemed 'irreversible' by doctors and specialists.[73] Incredibly, one well-regarded Masai traditional bonesetter believed that if an open fracture in the thigh (femur) of upper arm (humerus) had not healed completely in 8–10 days, the appendage had to be summarily amputated.[74] While we can date major limb amputations back to prehistoric times in the Babylonian "Code of Hammurabi" from 1700 BC, the operation has always been deemed the option of 'last resort' for surgeons worldwide.[75]

In Doumi's 2007, major amputation limb study in Western Sudan[75] revealed that of the 50 amputations, 96% of the limb losses were deemed 'potentially preventable', with sepsis accounting for the majority of amputations at 40%. These, and other imprudent decisions made by bonesetters without evidence-based medical knowledge and musculoskeletal diagnostic imaging support, bring about heart-rending, irreversible, life-changing, and/or life-threatening consequences to their unfortunate patients, who are oftentimes innocent children or teens [...] Some TBS patients pay for a single lapse in judgment with their very lives.

It is true that even with positive past experiences, there remain only a handful of people who relish the idea of undergoing a (potentially painful) dental appointment, surgical intervention, or doctor examination. Pain is, in fact, our body's best survival mechanism, and even though pain may prove incredibly uncomfortable, it remains the most effective mechanism for your brain to keep your body safe. Pain is useful and valuable. The language of pain, if you will, is the way your body speaks to you saying there's something terribly wrong here. For instance, bonesetter patients suffering from

Compartment Syndrome (too tight splinting) would do well to heed their increasingly agonizing pain—and listen to their body rebelling—warning against limb death, a lack of perfusion in their limb. For good or bad, corporeal discomfort is an integral part of the human condition and the only way we can mitigate pain is through restorative healing, therapeutic pain relief mechanisms, and good patient care. So, what constitutes 'good' patient care? Mainstream scholars and healthcare providers often point to "Picker's Eight Principles of Patient-Centered Care," which include: respect (involvement in decision making; cultural values, needs, and autonomy); coordination of care (ancillary, etc.); informed communication (progress, prognosis, processes of care); physical comfort; pain management; involvement of family and friends; continuity/post-discharge transition; and access to care.[76]

Hostility and Mistrust

Right or wrong, traditional African healers are ingrained as a deep-rooted and trusted community source of health information and treatment. Given proper skills and considerable patient oversight, they may prove a well-placed asset in combating Africa's trauma and infectious diseases. For instance, tuberculosis (TB) was on the rise in the Hlabisa district of KwaZulu/Natal, up by 360% in the seven years prior to 1999.[77] Interestingly, TB has a recognized, cost-effective, and readily available cure when patients comply with the set 6- to 8-month medical regimen. Due to the prolonged compliance period, there is a high drop-out rate among these highly contagious patients. In this study, traditional practitioners were trained to supervise and record the doses taken by each patient. "We were also taught about the symptoms of TB, so that when we pick them up in any of our other patients, we can refer people for a test,"[p89] said Jack Nyawuza, one of the 25 traditional healers who volunteered in the campaign.[77] Additionally, he said: "This information added to what we learn in our training as healers." Patients were delighted that the healers received this training: the healers lived nearby and could make home visits when patients were too sick to go to them. The results were quite notable, with traditional healers' patients reporting 89% program compliance (and two-thirds the overall mortality rate) when compared to 67% completion rate (under volunteer supervision).[77] The study noted that the healers seemed to welcome their newfound respect within the community.

Also, in a 2006 Nigerian study[8] conducted in Afuje and Ogua, a one-day training session for local bonesetters was conducted. The hands-on workshop in Afuje emphasized "safe conservative treatment of fractures,"[p3] focusing on diagnosis, patient selection (no open fractures), basic principles of fracture treatment, prevention of complications (transmission of infections), locally available referral services, and recorded outcomes). The secondary site, Ogua, was utilized as a 'control' (unaffected benchmark/point of comparison) and had no such TBS training sessions. The two-year study compiled (only) tibial shaft fractures.[8] In our opinion, this restriction was critically important to the study as it allowed a direct (and rather simplified) apples-to-apples comparison—decreasing the comorbidities of far more complex conditions associated with spinal, femoral (etc.) breaks—and omitting comorbidities of surrounding organ injuries, debris infection exposure, and/or blood loss from compound/open fractures, etc. The comparative Afuje-to-Ogua tibial fracture outcomes of Onuminya's 2006 study was as follows: a substantially high 19:5 ratio of 'acceptable union'; followed by a (contrary) 8:12 ratio of 'malunion'; a doubled rate 3:6 of 'nonunion'; an almost equal rate of 'delayed union' (7:8); a doubled rate of 2:5 of post-traumatic osteomyelitis; and finally, a quadrupled ratio of limb gangrene (100% resulting in amputations) of 1:4.[8] Onuminya further explains the study by noting the following: "[...] bonesetters have traditionally been considered secretive, and it was difficult to teach them how complications could be prevented"[8p322]; however, the significant increase in 'acceptable' unions was noticeably higher due to the 'infusion' of safe Western fracture care via these traditional Nigerian healing rituals and practices.

Yasin et al. reported that hospital congestion and the "hostile reception at public health care settings"[55p4] were determinants for seeking TBS care. Indeed, the global internet is flush with innumerable pieces of research pointing to the (general) disapproval of interactions with professional healthcare providers by many sub-Saharan African patients. Some of the hospital staff lack adequate training, and oftentimes refuse outright to give information to the patients about the nature of their ailments (either out of indifference, a fear of reprisal from the doctors, a dubious understanding of the patient's condition, or high workload, etc.). Many times, it is family or community members 'from the urban city' or an educated friend who will (ultimately) explain to the patient how Western-based hospital care can/has produced positive outcomes in similar cases, according to co-author Dr. Admasu, an Ethiopia-based orthopedic surgeon.

Delayed Presentation

Even when patients do not suffer an obvious fall, road traffic accident, work or sport mishap, any irregularities (lumps, swelling, inflammation, pain) in their bodily appendages can send them to TBS for a divination, incantation, treatment, or consultation. So, when poor, fearful, and/or medically illiterate patients develop soft tissue tumors, lesions in the skin of their legs or arms, etc., they may infer some type of some previous and/or forgotten minor injury. In Yongu et al. (2022) article: "Delayed Presentation of Bone and Soft Tissue Sarcoma of the Extremity in Makurdi: Do Traditional Bone Setters Play a Role?", Nigerian researchers reported significant patient presentation delays up to 14 weeks (46 weeks at patient presentation to hospital without TBS interventions versus 60 weeks with TBS regimen).[78] Several empirical studies reported the consultation of one (or more) traditional healers as the 'main cause' for delays, disruptions, and postponement(s) in appropriate patient care.[69,78,79,218]

Another study conducted in 2024 at the University of Hawassa in Ethiopia on 230 patients with musculoskeletal injury demonstrated that delayed presentation to a hospital is one of the factors associated with complications after traditional bonesetter treatment—lapses over 22.5 months post-injury showed a higher rate of complications (95 patients) when compared to under 22.5 month (only 49 patients).[63]

The late presentation of patients after seeking care from traditional bone setters can cause wide-ranging challenges to the orthopedic surgeon. These complications range from the psychosocial impacts of some treatment options to the demand for advanced (and not routinely accessible) treatment procedures. Amputations and complex limb deformity correction procedures are some examples. Additionally, some of the corrective orthopedic interventions require long-term commitments with repeated follow-up visits and radiographic imaging, which can lead to the economic bankruptcy and emotional frustration of patients.

The aforementioned 2024 report by Mengistu et al.[63] from the Hawassa University Comprehensive Specialized Hospital, Ethiopia, in contrast to other bonesetter studies, sought to uncover any gaps in orthodox health facilities that might drive patients towards TBS care. Over 230 post-TBS treatment patient interventions were studied, with 62% patients suffering some form of complication, including joint stiffness (30.4%), deformity (21.7%), skin sores/maceration (13.2%), malunion/nonunion (17%), chronic osteomyelitis and septicemia at 7.4%, gangrene and amputations at 2.3%, plus other issues such as muscle atrophy, Volkmann's Ischemic Contracture, etc.[63] The Ethiopian researchers deemed the number of complications among the trauma patients who first visited bonesetters as "unacceptably high," and in the multivariable logistic regression model, age of patients at <15 years or younger (adjusted odds ratio of 2.43, 95% CI = 1.21, 4.92), and a delayed hospital referral (adjusted odds ratio of 7.40, 95% CI = 3.86, 14.20) were correlated to complications (using binary logistic regression analysis, a 95% confidence interval, and a P-value <0.05).[63p47]

One 2018 study by Worku et al.[79] undertaken at Black Lion Hospital in Addis Ababa, attempted to address biases in TBS treatment. Even in this major capitol city, 84% of patients preferred TBS to the hospital for their initial treatment.[79] Approximately 25.9% of study's 227 patients believed that TBS was preferable to hospital care. Curiously, almost 60% also reported that they knew of specific drawbacks to utilizing traditional bonesetter care; however, of the studied trauma patients who said they were 'not knowledgeable' about TBS—they were almost 10 times (9.4×) more likely to prefer TBS.[79] In an urban city, Black Lion Hospital serves 340,000–400,000 patients annually, with the Adult Orthopedic ward 10,000—half of the patients suffering from acute fractures of the pelvis or upper and lower extremities (approx. 35–450 monthly).[79]

Traditional bone setters and healers also intervene in bone pathologies other than trauma such as bone and joint infection and bone tumors. These interventions lead to worsening of the disease and cause delay in presentation. It is quite common to see pathological fractures (i.e., fractures due to tumor) and infection being mismanaged in the traditional residential-home setting and this is mainly attributed to lack of understanding of disease pathology and progression, as well as a lack of radiographic and pathologic evidence (microscopic or macroscopic examination of diseased tissues, cells, or bodily fluids by a pathologist) to settle a diagnosis and tailor treatment.

In Nwachukwu et al. Nigeria-based research, one of the bonesetters explained that she tells all of her patients and their families to avoid Orthopedic centers because many of those who use such facilities return with 'missing legs' or with 'metal in their body'."[57] While 'mistrust' may remain the idiomatic reason for TBS patronage, it should, nonetheless, not be ignored. There is no dispute that amputations occur in hospital operating theaters—and not at the TBS residence(s). Contrarywise, from the public's 'distorted' and 'medically flawed' (weak in medical understanding or application) perspective, surgical-theater amputations have only ever occurred in the hospital, under a Western physician's care. And even though these medically necessary amputations—are indeed exacerbated by the bonesetters' machinations and the patient's delay in presentation to an orthopedic surgeon—these poor outcomes can be viewed as surreptitious political/social/tribal conspiracies, class hostilities, and even pure unadulterated money-making schemes by some patients and their families. There is also a generalized 'avoidance' of presenting to hospitals can stem from a fear of serious medical diagnosis, social stigma (AIDs, disabilities, amputees), medical distrust of health workers, long queues and delays in treatment (perceived or real), hospital bureaucracy, inadequate hospital beds, overcrowded bathrooms, etc., language barriers, and limited time with physicians.

All-Natural Remedies

Aside from the aforementioned 'determinants of patronage', some patients preferred the all-natural aspects of traditional remedies. Patients reported that the herbal-based remedies used by traditional healers were devoid of chemicals found in commercially sold tablets that can cause side effects.[80] Considering the leaps in modern twenty-first century medicine, it may seem nonsensical to choose botanical herbs on the basis of taste, appearance, or flavor properties, but they have been reported to be important selection criteria in traditional remedies.[47] Or as Zameer writes: "It is rather horrific that even in 21st century a lot of people do not know that there are no special herbs or spirit that draws and align fractures."[81p1]

Traditional healers tell community members that their remedies come from the soil—plants made by God himself. In fact, some TBS practitioners are known to canvass modern Western hospitals and clinics and "take away patients" with the "false promise that they can provide better care," that their brand of healing has no side effects, and that they can "cure all known diseases."[48p6] Other unscrupulous bonesetters convince their patients and family members that their fracture is "a condition not visible on X-rays"[p4] and that only they can administer the correct treatment.[82] Yet another study reported bonesetters telling people that "once you to the hospital, they will cut your leg"[68p4] (Participant 5, Orthopedist focus group). One of our informants, who was interviewed off the record, explained that she preferred herbal remedies due to their natural properties, and that they better aligned with her beliefs in holistic healing. She explained that while herbs remain her 'go-to-remedy', she acknowledges the importance of timely interventions in managing acute or persistent health problems.

According to Okaiyeto and Oguntibeju's 2021 study of African herbal medicines, the "ultraviolet rays in this region are stronger than those observed in other parts of the world, and this also enables the plants to accumulate some important bioactive substances"[p5988] of importance.[83] The same study[83] reported that "numerous African rural dwellers believe that since their ancestors used herbal mixtures/concoctions for their wellbeing in the past and with no side effect," the mixture's safety is guaranteed, "unfortunately, this assumption has led to several instances of organ damage and death of the users" as herbal components contain some bioactive compounds that are "potentially toxic."[p5988] Plus, due to a lack of temperature regulation (refrigeration at specified temperatures), post-harvest storage controls (such as ultraviolet light causing structural changes in the drug), and preservatives (that slow/stop the degradation; protect drugs from chemical change or microbial action), medicinal plants have shown "antibacterial and anti-inflammatory activity changes following storage, and is both species and temperature dependent,"p113 according to Fennell et al.[84]

"No Metal in My Body"

As with a preference for all-natural components in treatment, fracture patients also have stated that they do not want any foreign metal introduced (or implanted) in their body. As with anything unknown, the enigmatic metallurgical combinations used in today's high-tech implants and invasive traction devices pose a daunting challenge to those who prefer the physical insertion of (only) organic, non-artificial substances. As a valid counterargument, there have been innumerable reported people suffering from varieties of ingested, implanted, leaked, and bodily absorbed toxins via 'medical-grade' implants and devices (containing silicone, fillers, polypropylene chemicals, and heavy metal toxicity). In one study, post-implant patients reported not only body changes (inexplicable sickness, weakness), but also behavioral (anxiety, fear), and even psychological changes ("I feel like I have something foreign in my leg, psychologically I mean"p1), according to Tsalkitzi et al.[85]

Preferred 'Social Network'

Finally, we can attempt to calculate those 'unquantifiable' and indirect social determinants—like social support and community-held ideologies. Akakpo[60] argues that traditional bonesetters offer a "conducive, flexible, and very accommodating atmosphere," very much unlike Westernized hospitals "where care and management of fractures is the sole preserve of the hospital officials."p1375 The author goes on to state that the patient's family and community members provide encouragement and motivation for healing via "singing, storytelling, and playing of local games which serve as diversion therapy and pain-relieving mechanisms," all of which are social mechanisms that "support and hasten"p1375 the healing process.[60]

One of the critical concerns raised about 100% orthodox Western medical practice concerns that the treatment only addresses a patient's biological manifestation of illness, and makes no attempt to heal the patient's 'spirit'. During the end of the twentieth century, studies of religion and healing grew (one could argue that a new field was born) but in reality, the progression of the discipline simply confirmed the long-existing relationship between healers, patients, and religion—either as a private devotional practice or religion (in its broad institutional form). It is also the case that while traditional healing practices may not set up formal religious practices (led by hospital chaplains), religion is not ignored in traditional medical practices. It is common for a healer in Cameroon, for instance, to say that their work was specifically assigned (to them) by God. In some cases, the healers see their task as a calling from God or the ancestors (who are highly regarded as they have transitioned from this life and now live with other departed relatives, in close proximity to spiritual beings).

Specializations in Traditional Healing

We think that another fascinating insight that grew from this study was the notion of 'specialization' in traditional healing treatments. From our interviews and others, several practitioners listed off their 'area(s) of specialization'; in other words, they were recognized for particular illnesses, traumatic injuries, etc., and some practitioners refused to treat any and all issues. Our study has focused on the treatment of fractures, but for example, Pa Yerima Yongka treated many ailments in the Wimbum area, specializing in infertility. We must confess that the 'medical' diagnoses made by some traditional healers were, at best, dubious. As one example, a woman who was an asthmatic—was told she acquired the long-term inflammatory disease of the lung's airways—because she cried a lot as a baby (as opposed to viral respiratory infections, smoking, air pollution, morbid obesity, etc.). Other examples follow the various beliefs that infertility is caused by a living thing in the womb, an 'evil eye' curse, or a retribution from God or their 'fertility policing' ancestors (rather than male infertility, tubal obstructions, malnutrition, lifestyle behaviors, abortions, STDs, etc.). These challenges highlight the importance of understanding the education and personal history of healers. However, we should note that by the late 1970s (as was the case in some places in Cameroon), patients would derive a medical diagnosis from a trained physician, only to return home and seek healing by a traditional healer.

Noncompliance, Misconduct, and Negligence

Few researchers will argue the empirical, practical, and theoretical studies showing innumerable patient benefits from playing music, dancing, exercising, meditating, or undergoing hypnosis, chiropractic adjustments, biofeedback, or acupuncture (just to name a few). Indeed, some of these healing mechanisms show marked advances in decreasing anxiety, improving mental health, relieving pain, reducing inflammation, and boosting patient's immune response, etc. That being said, urgent life- or limb-threatening patient care is neither a democratic community-led meditation nor a sovereign familial contemplation. Any (willful and purposeful) misconduct, noncompliance, negligence, or circumnavigation of appropriate medical care is a disturbing overreach. Case in point: three of the four medical practitioners and coauthors Admasu, Flowers, and Richter have witnessed firsthand how easily this open, unrestricted, and 'shared' healing mindset can swiftly deteriorate into harmful family member overreach—causing the patient irreparable mis-/overdosing, misdiagnosis, provider neglect, and even the patient's untimely death. Several of these uncontrolled medical overreaches by (unlicensed nonmedical) friends, family, and community members Richter has witnessed firsthand include: the obstinate 'right to overdose' medications to hospitalized critical-care patients by family members (rationale: if one pill helps, then two will be even more helpful); a wanton 'right to disregard' healthcare staff and surrounding ward patients' public health welfare (via a refusal to don N-95 mask when diagnosed with highly communicable disease such as TB meningitis); a 'right to disruptive public behaviors' (witness to 18 visitors eating lunch at one patient's bedside in 'very urgent' orange hospital ward); a careless 'right to misuse and abuse' equipment, supplies, and charts belonging to the hospital; and finally, the unbelievably reckless 'right to treat without a medical license' gastrointestinal (GI-tube) feeding (with a bottle of open orange soda) and the adjustment of patient's IV medication and fluids by family members (rationale: more = better, so faster flow = better). Many of these incidents were marked first by a dereliction of duty by the assigned healthcare provider, followed by facility-wide negligence of hospital supervisors and administrators to enforce patient safety standards.

Ultimately, when we witness nurses and other healthcare providers willingly surrender their expert medical practices, procedures, and educational skills (dispense medications, record symptoms, operate medical equipment, etc.)—and publicly in a hospital setting—confer them to unwitting family members, these actions serve only to usurp a nurse's inherent value, sphere of influence, appreciation, systemic support, and respect. To wit: If an unskilled family member can perform these (skilled) nursing tasks, why is a nurse needed, and why should we invite her/his engagement in our family member's care? Nonetheless, patient safety and quality of care are essential components of any nation's nursing practice, and these priorities demand precision in order to deliver high-quality outcomes and patient-centered care. In the United States, by law via the American Nurses Association, RN tasks that "shall not be delegated are those that are inappropriate for a specific, unlicensed person" include those that require nursing judgment, critical thinking, or professional knowledge.[86] The tasks that registered nurses may never delegate include: medication administration (injection medications, except for insulin); sterile procedures (central line maintenance, tube feeding, wound care, and dressing changes); nursing assessment (problem identification, outcome evaluation, and counseling); client education (establishing outcomes and evaluating care); and nursing documentation processes (SOAPIE—Subjective, Objective, Assessment, Plan, Intervention, and Evaluation; ADPIE–Assessment, Diagnosis, Planning, Implementation, Evaluation; and DAR–Data, Action, and Response).[86]

As one example, nurses have an irreplaceable role and responsibility in medication administration, according to the NIH, in that they are "frequently the final person to check to see that the medication is correctly prescribed and dispensed before administration."[87p1] The five 'Nursing Rights of Medication Administration' (in the traditional sequence) include: 1) 'Right patient'—the correct recipient for whom medication was prescribed; 2) 'Right drug'—checking expiration date, patient allergies, brand and generic name(s) so no medical errors due to misreading letters or numerals; 3) 'Right Route'—oral, intramuscular, intravenous (IV), topical, subcutaneous injection, central venous catheter, patient-controlled analgesia (PCA), epidural infusions, and intrathecal administration; 4) 'Right time'—in order to maintain a therapeutic effect or level; and 5) 'Right dose'—check on correct dosage, conversion of units, and substance concentration. Medical errors and Adverse Drug Effects (ADEs) qualify as "unintended injuries or insults directly related to medical interventions involving a drug," according to the NIH, "resulting in disability at discharge, death, or extended hospital stay that is the result of health care management rather than by the patient's underlying disease process."[87p1] As we can see, so much can go wrong so quickly in medication administration.

Richter vividly recalls one Ethiopian daughter who had overstayed the visitor's 'Red Zone' ICU patient allotment (one adult visitor per patient) at the University of Gondar's Hospital. When asked to leave the ward, the irate (unlicensed nonmedical) daughter turned around vehemently and loudly shouted at Richter: "Fine! You take of her now!" Well, yes indeed, it is, in fact, the role of healthcare providers to provide all care necessary while the patient is remanded to a hospital ward—and, most especially, while the patient is admitted within a 'Red', ICU, or Critical Care zone. The unspoken license of family members to care for any acutely ill patient smacks of healthcare provider malpractice (as they knowingly and deliberately abdicate their patient responsibilities) to an unwitting spouse, son, daughter, or naïve visitor who may become an innocent actor involved in the patient's deterioration or death.

So, when patient's family members—who have zero training in sterility, medication dosages, IV drip rates, GI tube feeding, etc.—are freely given the unsafe task(s) of invasive and life-altering care, they can play a duped culprit in the patient's injury, disability, or death. If we only examine a single witnessed (nonmedical) family member overreach, the GI-tube feeding, we can find a litany of complications from unsterile practices, including, but not limited to: bleeding, infection, tube breakage/knotting/leakage/obstruction, necrotizing fasciitis, peritonitis, accidental tube removal, ulceration, and many, many more conditions. It is important to note that healthcare providers and doctors undergo extensive training in medical science, diagnosis, and treatment (which most family members do not have) and that family members commonly have some emotional bias in a given situation (either via social media, personal experience, or unproductive WebMD searches) which can muddy unbiased judgment(s). In the end, the importance of a 'checks-and-balances' collaboration—with the healthcare provider making medical diagnosis and providing hands-on care, and the patient and family involved in discussions of possible treatment options—remains paramount to every patient's best outcome.

Scarcity in Credible Accounts

Due to the often unrestricted and/or unregulated nature of TBS practices, there are "no reliable statistics to gauge the number of patients attended to by indigenous Orthopedic healers," stated Taylor.[88p263] Even with a global literature review of traditional bone-setting mechanisms, patient treatment options, clinically assessed complications, and/or outcomes, there remains little standardization and/or global data consensus to be found in credible academic journals. However, credible published hard-science journal articles do exist, and they are led primarily by Nigerian, Ghanaian, Ethiopian, Indian, Sudanese, as well as a handful of other LMIC scholars.

That being said, a global TBS literature meta-search review shows published academic studies in PubMed, Embase, ScienceDirect, SCOPUS (with patient outcomes) starting in approximately 1986 in China.[89] For purposes of this study, we reviewed over 27 articles that showed clinically proven (via imaging diagnostics) medical outcomes, including acceptable or non-acceptable/malunion, deformities, permanent nerve injuries, limb shortening, paralysis, infections, etc. The preponderance of clinical studies we assessed came from Nigeria, with a total of 9 from Nigeria: (northern region in 1999; southwest in 2001; southwestern region in 2004; 2005; two in 2006 (Afuje site A and Ogu site B); 2011; northcentral in 2013; and one literature review of 176 bone-setting studies published by Ndubuisi O. Onyemaechi in 2021,[90] and more. Our three chosen studies from India were published in 2015 and 2017, as well as Ethiopia (southern region in 2013, southern region in 2014, pediatric study in 2018, and northwest in 2022), and more. We also cite two studies from each of the following two countries of Pakistan (2012 and 2018) and Sudan (2009 and 2010). Other solo regional studies, just to name a few, hailed from Bangladesh (2013), China (1986), northern Ghana (2013), Indonesia (2018), northern Tanzania (2021), Turkey (2015), and one literature review of 12 published TBS studies out of the United Kingdom.[91]

As the 27 specified published articles bear no standardization of their stated protocols (mechanism(s) of injury, etc.), TBS treatments, imaging, patient groups (pediatric or adult), or organization of possible outcomes—this is a questionable apples-to-oranges comparison, however, it endeavors to begin to quantify the personal (corporal pain, and oftentimes unnecessary suffering), socioeconomic (long-term disabilities, permanent nerve injury, deformities, paralysis), and professional costs (high-acuity orthopedic and/or infection care, surgical interventions, and prosthetic specialties) of global traditional bonesetter complications that have, in fact, been clinically diagnosed and documented.

Bonesetters in Modern Literature and Historical Works

And while, at this current time, we may be hard-pressed to locate data concerning positive, unbiased, medically authenticated (scholarly) patient outcomes—due to inherent secrecy, poor data collection, and a general lack of mutual pan-African collegial collaboration(s)—some, albeit earlier manuscripts, and historical, romanticized, and fictional literary accounts do exist. Three published commercial books we decided to include in this manuscript (due to their historical and cultural insights), are the following: "That Bonesetter Woman"[92] from 2022, "In the Bonesetter's Waiting Room: Travels through Indian Medicine"[93] from 2016; and Amy Tan's more-recent 2001 bestseller, "The Bonesetter's Daughter,"[94] which is based on a true story.

In Frances Quinn's historical fiction "That Bonesetter Woman," there is a main character that wishes to follow in her father's footsteps as a bonesetter.[92] However, the novel is set in 1757 Georgian London, and the character is a female, so she is unable to even assist her father's (very successful) medical practice. Though irrefutably a work of fiction, the historical novel does serve to entertainingly dramatize the rather vicious name-calling, slanderous abuse, and open animosity that played out in public forums, placards, and newspapers between physicians and bonesetters at that time. The physicians were (literally) fighting for their livelihoods and to keep their burgeoning professional disciplines and accreditations collectively intact. Interestingly, the village farrier—who trimmed horses' shoes—remained, in fact, the cheapest option at that time for splinting and setting human fractures.[92]

Prasad's book primarily plots a path that helps explain the incredibly diverse history of India's seven-tiered healthcare system.[93] These officially recognized and utilized types of healthcare, according to Prasad, include: English (a.k.a. Western, biomedicine, allopathic, or modern); Ayurveda; Yoga; Siddha; Unani (Greek via Arab influence); and then, nineteenth-century European-based Naturopathy, or Homeopathy.[93] The sextet acronym 'AYUSH' is often used as a collective term for these systems which serves up to 70% of the population; it mirrors a Sanskrit word meaning 'long life'.[92] It is remarkable to note that not one, but seven types of healthcare, are officially recognized, licensed, promoted, respected, and (legally) accepted as 'beneficial' by a single nation. This enormous amount of choice, while daunting in its scope and myriad(s) of regulated protocols, seemingly attempts to honor disparate cultural understandings of approaches to injury care, as well as disease and its prevention. Such a huge national panorama of healthcare choices can be viewed as a regulatory nightmare, fiscal folly, and so on—or rather an ingenious integration of ancient cultural traditions with cutting-edge medical technological developments—with neither one considered the lesser.

Like Prasad, John M. Janzen describes patterns of 'medical pluralism' in healings among the BaKongo of Lower Zaire in Africa in his 1978 book "The Quest for Therapy in Lower Zaire," which reviews real-life cases and on-the-ground ethnographical contexts to explore what social transactions, decision making, illnesses, and resource allocations are used in the choice of therapy between 'cosmopolitan medicine' and traditional healing practices.[22] In the book, Central Africans show how differently designed and conceived medical systems can, and do, mutually coexist. Conversely, "when the characterization of African and other health systems" is deemed as supernatural, it "becomes a rationale for making no effort to understand, let alone accommodate, existing biomedical beliefs."[95p218]

Amy Tan's "The Bonesetter's Daughter" (2001) is of interest in that the Chinese bonesetter's family members cannot verbatim pass down the father's wisdom to the main character—but she is given an 'oracle bone' (which they also refer to as 'dragon bones'), a symbolic token of the entitlement to her rightful lineage of bonesetters.[94] These 'bones' hold tremendous spiritual power as they (physically retain) and store ancient curses, which serve as modern-day harbingers of anxieties.[94] Interestingly, this novel does give a nod to the real historical account of the 'Peking Man' (prehistoric species *Homo erectus*, a species of archaic human) excavation in 1927.[94] The author utilizes the true event as an interesting backdrop to explain the recognized fiscal and supernatural value of these so-called 'dragon bones'.

Also bearing mention include one seventeenth century work, "The Compleat Bone-Setter" by Friar Moulton in 1656[96]; and two nineteenth century manuscripts entitled: "The Art of the Bonesetter" by George W. Bennett in 1884[97]; and "On bone-setting (so called), and its relation to the treatment of joints crippled by injury, rheumatism, inflammation" by PH Wharton in 1871.[98] These three accounts help to shed light on bonesetters' very little-known (earlier) American and English methods, their impacted communities, and their (oftentimes disgruntled) surgical counterparts.

To begin with, is Moulton's aptly (but rather extensive) entitled 1656 book: "The *compleat* [sic] bone-setter: wherein the method of curing broken bones, and strains, and dislocated *joynts* [sic], together with ruptures, vulgarly called broken *bellyes* [sic], is fully demonstrated. Whereunto is added *The* perfect oculist, and *The mirrour* of health, treating of the pestilence, and all other diseases incident to men, women and children. Also, the acute judgement of urines". This manuscript marks the one of the scholarly beginnings of documenting bonesetter methods for fractures, dislocations, and sprains.[96]

Then, George Matthews Bennet's 1884 manuscript illustrates how he himself was a former (successful) patient of a bonesetter, as well as a practicing bonesetter in England. Bennett broke his leg as a child and was treated by a bonesetter, so he describes his treatment by the local bonesetter. He also gives a comprehensive cultural perspective of his time and the historical perception on the practice of bone-setting and traditional medicine. The initial chapters take the reader through his painful recovery processes and impact(s) from the fracture on his young life.[97] Bennett then spends the remainder of his manuscript vindicating bonesetters as legitimate and effective practitioners, despite society's surrounding skepticism and criticism (primarily pushed via the current medical establishment). Throughout the book, Bennett argues that bone-setting is a valuable service, and that there are numerous examples of successful treatments and recoveries—that have been disregarded and disparaged through a 'knowledge bias' through the machinations of the United States. Though he asserts his so-called 'vindication' of TBS; he does acknowledge that during his medical tenure that there was a lack of recorded cures and that bone-setting was "arts of the charlatan and the quack."[97pviii]

Sex-Disaggregated Data in Traditional Bone-Setting

As Dr. Marianne J. Legato explains the ad hoc 'gender irrelevancy' (interchangeability) in the medical field: "Unless they are focusing on the reproductive system, most doctors have a tendency to treat patients as though were all the same sex: Male."[99pl] At first blush, researchers may not deem sex-disaggregated data to be a compelling issue in traditional African fracture care. However, as in most gender-based, socioeconomic and biological variances cases, a patient's biological sex should, indeed, routinely be considered. So, we will start with the obvious differences in sex-disaggregated patient numbers, which was found to be substantial in the vast majority of studies.

When patients with complications finally decide to seek Western biomedical care, it is interesting to note that some complications are more accepted by the society than others—disturbingly, complications (such as deformities, poor gait, etc.) in children and women are disregarded more frequently than those in men, according to Dr. Admasu's experiences in Ethiopia. In Ghana, Dr. Dominic Konadu-Yeboah, who serves as AO Alliance faculty and is head of trauma and orthopedics at Komfo Anokye Teaching Hospital (KATH) in Kumasi, Ghana, had this to say: "The rate of traditional bonesetter-related limb gangrene, disability, infections, and death in Ghana is alarming, particularly among children."[9p1]

Sex and Gender: Biological Issues

From the outset (when sex-disaggregated data were available), meta-data analyses showed a preponderance of male trauma (fracture care) patients. As stated succinctly by Ewuoso et al., the utilization of TBH is highest among men under 37 years of age in their "productive years" who are the "economic lifeline of any society."[48p7] A few examples of sex-disaggregated TBS fracture male-to-female patient ratios include: 68% male prevalence[56,100]; a 3:1 sex ratio among pediatric limb amputation patients[55]; a 60% male cohort of patients[73]; and in Udosen et al. (2006) study from Nigeria, there was a 4:1 male/female ratio of the clients.[101] However, a study from India showed an ever-so-slight 'role reversal' in sex-based patients, with a 14:16 male-to-female ratio among patients in Ananthapuramu.[93]

In Yongu et al.'s (2022) article: "Delayed Presentation of Bone and Soft Tissue Sarcoma of the Extremity in Makurdi: Do Traditional Bone Setters Play a Role?", researchers found that their Nigerian female patients exhibited a significantly longer delay in care-seeking behavior when compared to their male counterparts, primarily attributed to lower financial and social status, as well as overall family caregiver/sole provider role(s).[78]

Which all begs the question, of course: How is sex-disaggregated data relevant when studying Traditional Bone Setting (TBS) practices? First, we will address sex-based differences—those based in (anatomical) physiological, toxicological, and/or pharmacological bases, then we will unpack the wide variety of gender-based issues in TBS, which are rooted in social, religious, educational, and other 'self-determination' dynamics. So, as for physiological differences, we can go to 'gender-based biology' which "identifies physiological and biological differences between men and women at the subcellular, cellular, tissue, organ, and system level, and the effects of pharmaceutical agents."[102pix] For the purposes of this study, we will attempt to refine those differences that may well be relevant to fracture care, blood flow, infection rates, and outcomes. As Langley states, overall "women tend to have greater bio-availability and slower clearance of drugs" when compared to men, and the consequence of this is that the "correct doses in males may be relatively higher for females."[102p308] For instance, studies have found a significant "28%–36% decrease in the rate of gastric emptying" in pre-menstrual females (308); male-to-female ratios of post-surgical infections are 1.5:1; and post-traumatic sepsis rates occur more in males (at 31%) than females (17%).[102p247]

In collective terms, studies show men and women have (significant) differences in their immune systems (autoimmune diseases higher in women), hormone production (men produce 52% more serotonin needed to prevent depression), the 'pharmacokinetics' of drugs, and metabolism. Sex-based differences in pharmacokinetics—a study of how the body absorbs, distributes, and eliminates medicines—is basely largely on our differing metabolism in our gastrointestinal tracts. In general terms: women have less acid in their stomach (i.e., less ulcers) and slower digestion times (33 vs. 47 hours); women have a longer colon (by about 10 centimeters); women have more body fat (18%–20% vs. 10%–15% of their body weight, respectively); less body water content (55% vs. 60%); and slower emptying times (except in the middle of the menstrual cycle, when speed increases).[99,102,103] Therefore, considering these conflicting physical structures and biochemical makeups, it would only stand to reason that there are, indeed, sex-based differences in pharmacokinetic studies that can potentially affect fracture treatment and outcomes. In fact, some 70% of all injury-related orthopedic patients comprise male patients (compared to 55% female)[102]—with young men and old females making up the groups 'most likely' to visit an orthopedic specialist, according to Langley. So, when fracture care is provided, these physiological differences should be considered. As for prescribing antibiotics and anti-inflammatory for fracture patients, studies confirm that females clear several medications from their systems faster than men (due to CYP 3A4 enzyme system up to 40% more active in females), which include antibiotics like Erythromycin, steroids like Prednisolone, Calcium channel-blockers (Verapamil), and sedatives (like Valium, or generic Daizepam).[99] It is interesting to note that despite these well-known evidence-based differences between men and women, "sex-specific dosing recommendations are absent for most drugs,"[103p43] according to University of California's Riverside Pharmacology Professor Chu.

Gender-Based Issues

We will now refocus our physiological sex differences to gender-based issues in fracture care. Here, we can unpack a very wide variety of psychosocial, environmental, and cultural factors. Gender-based explanations on fracture care procurement, TBS usage, assessment, treatment, and outcome can perhaps be categorized via theses six pre-defined categories: behavioral (risk-taking characteristics), sociological (self-determination), occupational, economical, recreational, and genetic/hereditary (osteoporosis, autism, etc.).

First of all, behavioral issues can include everything from smoking and drinking to (general overall) aversion to (or penchant for) a variety of risk-appetites. Generally speaking, female drivers are involved (statistically) in fewer alcohol-related crashes; however, women that are arrested for drunk driving are more likely to suffer traumatic injuries with higher rates of major amputations. In Doumi's Western Sudan study, for example, the male-to-female ratio of amputations was 75%–25%, respectively.[75] Again, the study noted that patients presenting with gangrenous limbs had "post-fracture manipulations and tight inappropriate splintage by traditional bonesetters."[75p238] As for gender differences, this particular aforementioned study reported that perhaps male patients were more prone to vascular atheromatous diseases due to cigarette smoking habits,[75] a habit which has deleterious effects on the body's healing process.

Second, sociological inequities can account for females not having access to (or a choice) involving their healthcare due to their low social power, religious constraints (such as female only physicians), lack of financial security. Back in the 1960s, Johan Galtung first coined the term "structural violence" as "unequal life chances"—or "avoidable impairment of fundamental human needs"—that usher in inequitable access to resources, political power, education, healthcare, or legal status.[104p170] As Galtung so eloquently stated: "There may not be any person who directly harms another person in the structure. The violence is built into the structure and shows up in unequal power and consequently as unequal life chances [...]."[104p171] When we evaluate feminist discourse(s) within the decision-making paradigm of TBS care, we clearly observe some controlling constructs of misogyny, ageism, anti-feminist, and patriarchal authority in place. It is this structural violence, according to Richter et al., that "fabricates pronounced and preventable causes of premature death, suffering, unnecessary disabilities, as well as the exacerbation of lower acuity illnesses/diseases into higher acuity illnesses/disease phases."[28p97] The time-lapse of patient care between the (initial low-acuity) application of an improper TBS splint (causing Compartment Syndrome)—to the late-stage, high-acuity intervention of surgical treatment illustrates how constraints and patriarchal/familial subordination in untimely decisions can lead to unnecessary suffering, limb loss, and even death for women. Third, occupational differences include more men working outside the home and driving "more miles per year than females."[102p324] As a fourth category, fiscal concerns reflect that women (globally) only control 32% of the world's wealth (primarily in the United States and other developed areas), while comprising half of the world's population (4.10 billion males at 50.28% vs. 4.06 billion at 49.72%),[105] according to the UN World Population Prospects in 2024.

Our final category, genetic or hereditary differences only come into our purview due to issues such as osteoporosis (female-to-male ratio in bone density loss is 2:1); osteoporosis-related fractures occur in 50% females, but only 20% of males over the age of 65.[102] It is interesting to note that the risk of fractures among young males is higher than females—until they reach the age of 45—when the sex-based ratios, in an extraordinary reversal of fortune, flip-flop their fracture rankings.

While we conclude our discussions on sex-disaggregated data, we can also interject a quick note on age-disaggregated data here. Pediatric cases were not included in this study as children are rarely, if ever, considered the primary decision-makers in obtaining TBS care in Africa. In Yasin et al.'s research concerning pediatric limb amputations and the role of traditional Ethiopian '*wogesha*' (bonesetter), the most common indication among children at 55.5% was gangrene "arising from treatment of limb injuries by traditional bone-setters."[55p2] Yasin et al. went on to report that all the causes for amputation are "non-communicable conditions," concluding that the majority of amputations "could have been prevented" through "health education, early patient presentation, and appropriate treatment in a modern health facility."[55p1]

Surely, the genesis of expanding and exploiting our female sex-/gender-based physiological and behavioral differences in contrast to men is not a matter of 'political correctness', some elitist 'woke' agenda, or publishable feminist angst. It is, indeed, as Legato summarizes it, an "intellectual imperative."[99p241] And this intellectual imperative is one of the most powerful tools we have to (both) correct and expand our knowledge of human pain management, disaster decision-making behaviors, disease prevention, as well as disability and injury risk-reduction strategies. In the following chapter, we will allow traditional bonesetters, their patients, and orthopedic surgeons who treat post-TBS patients—to speak directly to their global contemporaries.

Chapter 3

IN THEIR OWN WORDS: CONVERSATIONS WITH WORKING AFRICAN BONESETTERS, THEIR PATIENTS, AND THE MEDICAL PRACTITIONERS WHO TREAT THEM

While the auspices of bonesetter practices are veiled in secrecy—locally restricted rituals, unidentified ingested mixtures, secret poultice concoctions, forbidden authority, supernatural skills, exclusive privileges, and birthrights, etc.—these critical one-on-one interviews strive to 'lift the veil' off this secretive community and lay bare their practices, beliefs, and/or materials that comprise their work. Many bonesetters acknowledge an 'inherited profession' of family, also known as "the tendency for children to enter the same or similar occupations as their parents," according to the Sociology Dictionary.[106] The knowledge of African bone-setting is oftentimes verbally passed from one generation to another, without any resort to formal (written or recorded) documentation. Techniques are passed on from generation to generation or are personally discovered (anew) through trial-and-error practice. Through the practice of apprenticeship and on the job training, traditional bonesetters "pass down the knowledge of bone manipulation, herbal topical applications and sometimes oral ingestions to the next generation, often consisting of family members."[107p81] And, although we do not know the denominator (i.e., how many people are successfully treated by the TBS), we can almost immediately recognize the obvious physiological pathologies of malunion, contractures, osteomyelitis, limb shortening, etc.

Of the eight ensuing interviewed bonesetters for this study, we include: four Ghanaian TBS (4 males), one Ethiopian TBS (1 male), one Cameroonian TBS (1 male), and two Zimbabwean TBS (1 female and 1 male). In Ghana, one TBS lived in the (central) Kintampo area, one in a small town on the Kintampo-Tamale Road (approximately a 30-minute drive from Kintampo), with the third and fourth bonesetters worked in the pastoral village of Nkoranza, Ghana. In Ethiopia, our male TBS worked in the urban setting of Addis Ababa. In Zimbabwe, our male TBS lived in the Masvingo Province, and the only female TBS we were able to interview resided in the Midlands Province (Gokwe Nembudziya). The interview with our Cameroonian bonesetter, Pa Tamnjong, working in Ntumbaw Village, can be read in Chapter 1. For more a detailed identification of these aforementioned geographic regions, see Figure 1.1 (map of Africa); Figure 1.2 (map of Cameroon with locations); Figure 1.3 (map of Ethiopia with locations); Figure 1.4 (map of Ghana with locations); and Figure 1.5 (map of Zimbabwe with locations).

IN THEIR OWN WORDS: Agyemin Boateng Daniel, 60, Bonesetter, Ghana

Again, of our four selected Ghanaian bonesetters, one lived in the (central) Kintampo area, one in a small town on the Kintampo-Tamale Road (approximately a 30-minute drive from Kintampo), and the third and fourth bonesetters worked in the village of Nkoranza, approximately a two-hour drive from Kintampo. These Ghanaian bonesetters practice "apra aduro" (or 'injury medicine' in local Twi language) care based on long-established cultural practices; however, the safety and efficacy of traditional methods are sparsely evaluated via modern Western medical diagnostic imaging techniques (X-rays, CT scan, MRI, etc.).

Like his father and grandfather before him, Agyemin Boateng Daniel, is a bonesetter (in 2016 age 60) living in the rural town of Asuano, Ghana. In his native Twi language, Daniel explained that he uses 'aduro' (herbal medicine) for 'apra' (injuries). His 'aduro' consists primarily of two types of ground bark from the Badie tree. Daniel said he knows when a patient has 'a broken bone when their leg or hand is [flapping] shaking wrong'. He then is able to palpate the location of the fracture, but some people do bring him their X-rays from a clinic or hospital, and he likes holding the X-rays up the light to view bone configurations.

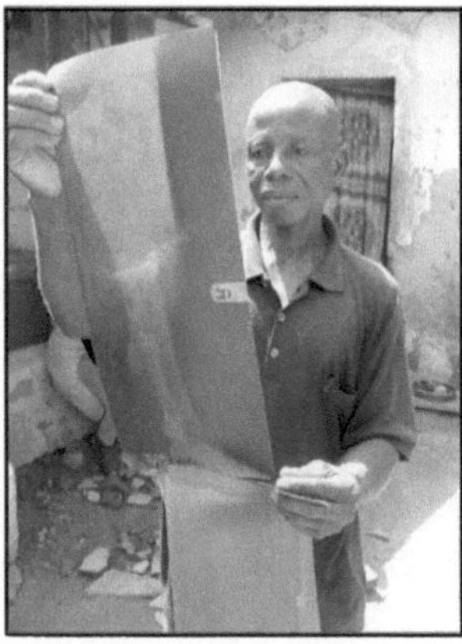

"I know it is a broken bone when their leg or hand is [mimics flapping motion] shaking wrong…

If the bone is out, we push it back into the skin. If we cannot put it back in, we say to go to the hospital."

- *Agyemin Boateng Daniel, 60*

Photo 3.1. We show Agyemin Boateng Daniel some X-rays of various fractures. He acknowledged having looked at some X-rays from his patients before.

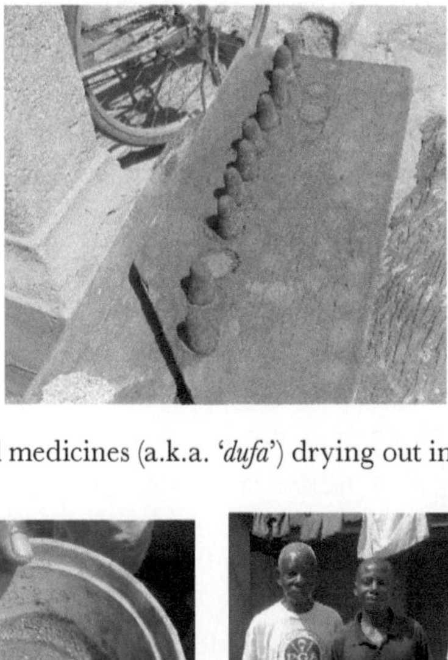

Photo 3.2. His herbal medicines (a.k.a. '*dufa*') drying out in the sun.

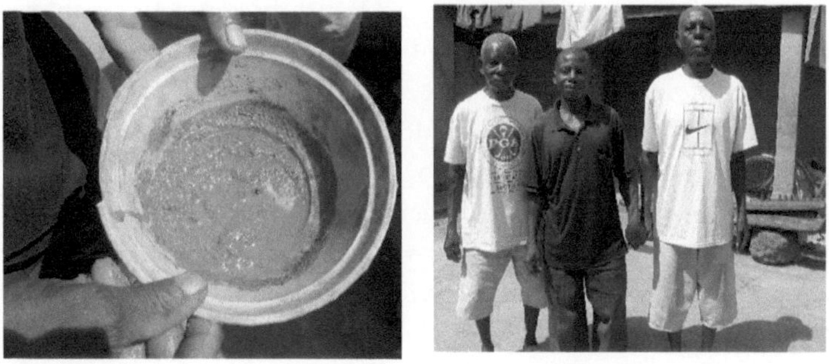

Photo 3.3–3.4. (L) Daniel showing his well-known '*dufa*' which he applies to injuries. '*Dufa*' is a Twi term that translates to an herbal remedy, whereby various ingredients are pounded and dried into hard round/rectangular shapes; it is used for treating assorted ailments and (also) as a protection against witchcraft in Ghana. Daniel creates his paste by mixing together handfuls of water and crushed ginger nut, roots from the Badie tree, and wisa (West African black peper). (R) Daniel flanked by his grandfather and father.

According to Daniel, when a patient comes to him for fracture care, he begins by boiling a large vat of water over the fire. He then 'massages' the fracture with a towel that has been soaked in the hot water. Daniel explains that to some people, hot water is an "abomination"—a traditional belief that some Akan/Ghanaian people have whereby people will break out in a bodily rash or have an allergic reaction to hot water. Therefore, if the patient refuses Daniel's use of hot water, he agrees to use tepid/room temperature water. Speaking of which, it is worthwhile to note that water holds a deep and indelible place in Ghanian spirituality.[200] This reverence in the use of water for healing is illustrated through the local Ghanian Akan proverb says, "When the chicken drinks water, it shows it to God"[108pl] (or '*Akoko nom nsu a, odze kyere Nyame*' in Twi language), as the chicken must raise its head up to the sky in order to drink, according to Hagan's piece entitled: "Water and Spirituality in Some African Cultures and Traditions."[108] However, in some rural Ghanaian societies, the practice of drinking and/or utilizing hot, boiled water 'spoils' it for human use, and/or makes it unpalatable. Richter and Flowers experienced this over and over during their medical services to help eradicate guinea worm (*Dracunculus medinensis*) parasitic infections with World Missions Possible (www.worldmissionspossible.org) in northern Ghana—whereby efforts to teach local residents in N'gani and Yendi to boil contaminated river water were consistently stymied. It should be noted here that Sture Lagercrantz reported very similar practices in Tunisia, Algeria, Morocco, The Gambia, and Senegal, whereby fabric compresses are moistened with cold water (sometimes infused with kola leaves) and an 'energetic massage' is applied among the Diola, the Futa (or Fouta) Djallon, the Malinke, and Maninka people.[74]

The bonesetter will then apply his *dufa* paste fresh every day over the open or closed fracture. After much prodding, Daniel disclosed all six ingredients he uses to make his *dufa*. While some bonesetters might be willing to share some of the ingredients, an 'exact' list of ingredients is considered a solemn tradesman's secret. In Blesching's 2018 blog, she spoke with a Ghanaian bonesetter in Tema who was quick to point out that "too many times the white man has come and stole medicinal knowledge, made billions, and shared none of it with those who discovered and generously shared them in the first place."[109pl] However, we will only disclose half (three of the six) trees, plants, and herbs Daniel utilized: Badie—the Badie tree (*Bridelia ferruginea*); Kankan—fermented black garlic (*Allium sativum*); and Aboboma—also known as wild soursop or wild African custard-apple (*Annona senegalensis*). He then heats plantain leaves over an open fire in his familial compound, making the leaves smooth and pliable. Once the leaves are ready, he binds the fracture with the leaves and then applies a bamboo splint. These will be discussed in more detail in Chapter 4.

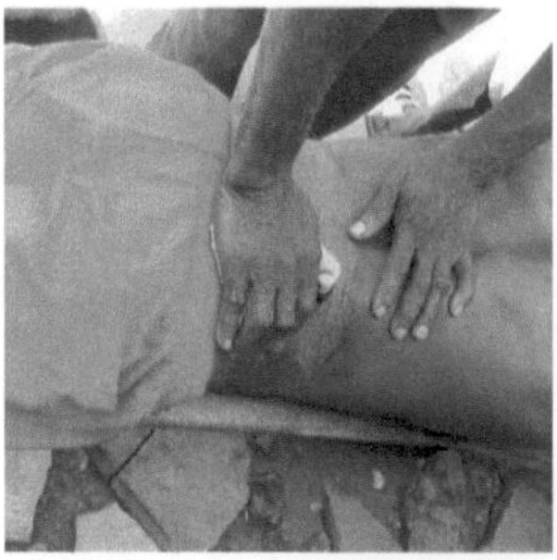

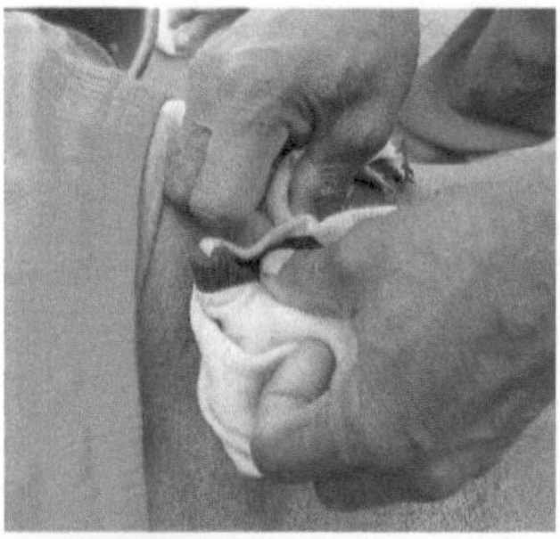

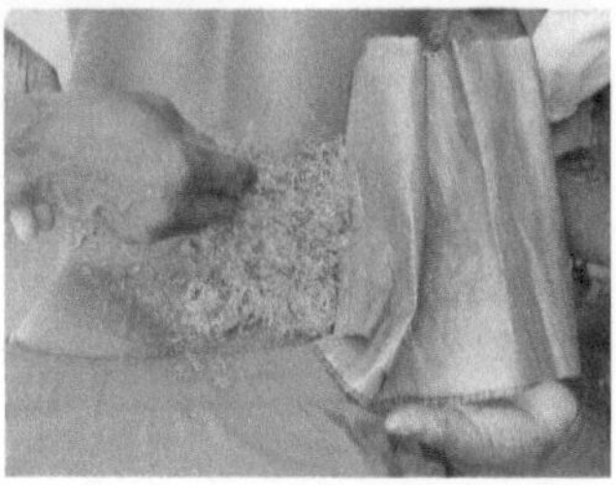

Photo 3.5–3.7. (Upper L) Daniel massages his patient's injured back. (Upper R) Daniel prefers to use hot water for the massages, unless the patient refuses it as hot (or even warm) water is considered by some villagers as an 'abomination'. (Above) Daniel applies his herbal medicines to patient's back.

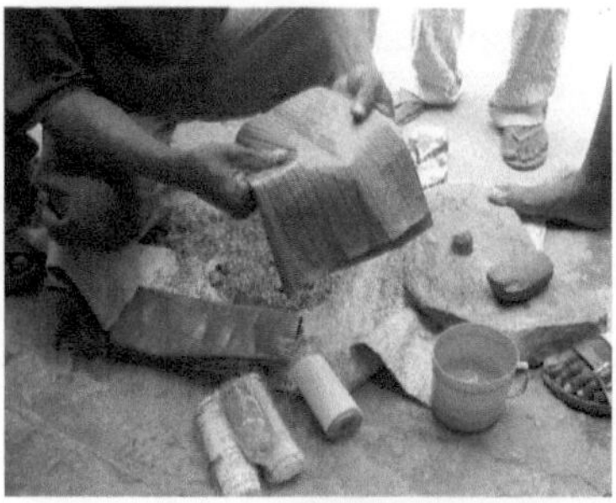

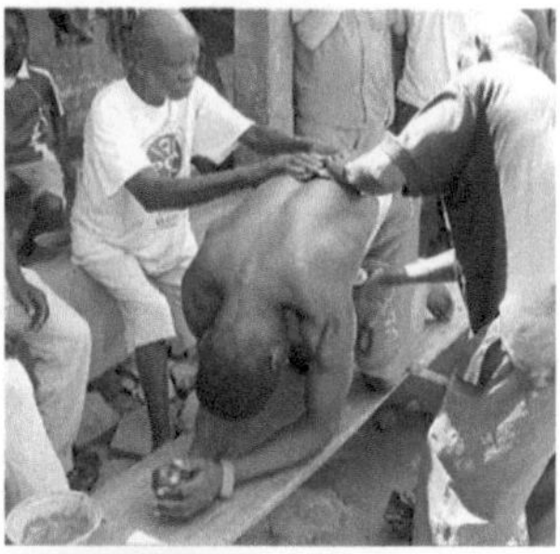

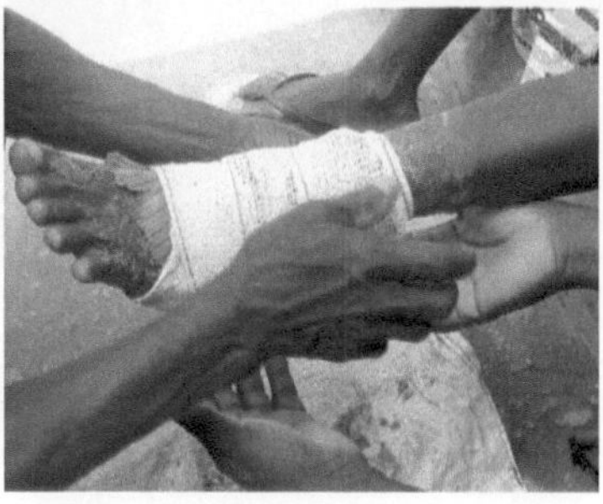

Photo 3.7–3.9. (Top) Daniel shows all of his supplies used in injury management. (Middle) Daniel and his grandfather apply bandages to back injury. (Bottom) Daniel treating patient with ankle injury.

The traditional bonesetter explained that sometimes they will push an open compound fracture bone "back into the skin," but if they see that they cannot put it back in, they tell the patient they should go and get surgery. As for pain, Daniel shakes his head saying: "In three days the pain will be gone," but the patient can purchase aspirin from the neighboring city if they are interested in additional pain relief. The cost for Daniel's service ranges from 100 to 400 *Ghanaian cedis* (approximately $17—$68 USD using November 2020 exchange rate of 1 USD = 5.8 cedis). Each patient is responsible for bring their own bandages which they can buy new from a neighboring city pharmacy or purchase used bandages in the local area. On average, patients remain under the bonesetter's care for four to nine weeks. Daniel explains that it takes "three good months" of no walking on a fractured leg as the "bone is joining."

"We like the injury at the moment when it happens. But some people wait a long time before they come. Then the patient will need to have the bone broken again and fixed. We won't break it even though the patient will prefer, but we will not do it," said Daniel.

IN THEIR OWN WORDS: Robert Fosu Appiah, Bonesetter, 56, Ghana

Robert Fosu Appiah, (in 2016 age 56), stated that he had gone through five years of training before becoming a bonesetter. "Traditional bonesetters are not many," he said, "Others should continue their studies rather than to try and help other people. I get my power from God." Appiah lives in the Brahoho (Nkoranza district) of Ghana. "It's from the medicine. You can get to know the medicine [the herbal recipe], but if you don't go through the process, you will not get the medicine correct. The skills in applying the medicine are also the power," Appiah explained.

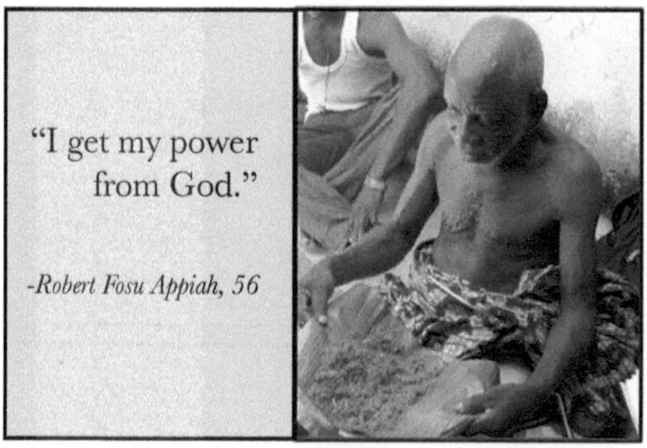

Photo 3.10. Despite the bonesetter keeping all ingredients a 'trade secret', TBS patients (like the one pictured above) set their trust and beliefs in the bonesetters' generational training, spiritual powers, and local ethnobotanical wisdom.

Appiah uses *Kyerebenteme*—bark and leaves; *Sunontokwa kofoo* (elephant fighter)—leaves only; *Brepuu*—roots; and *Jam wisa* (local black pepper). He explained that you then must have one day to let the bark, roots, and the leaves dry completely, then you add water to the mix, forming a paste. The paste then remains on the bone for three days. Appiah explained that the paste and the drink [potion] work "together"—both symbiotically and simultaneously.

IN THEIR OWN WORDS: Ayele Mengistu, 75, Bonesetter, Ethiopia

Ayele Mengistu practices bone-setting in the capital city of Ethiopia, Addis Ababa. At 75 (in 2023), he boasts some 50 years of experience, managing his own private practice over the past 12 years. Over his five decades of practice, he received training from three separate fields of fracture care: sports, medicine, and traditional African bone-setting. Mengistu stated that he completed Sport Federation (Ethiopian Athletics Federation)[204], medical training, and traditional training passed down from his maternal grandmother. We can refer to Mengistu as a 'tradorthopedic', a term first coined by Onuminya in her 2006 article entitled: 'Performance of a trained traditional bonesetter in primary fracture care'.[8] Mengistu utilizes (some) facets of modern diagnostics, has received some formal 1st Aid and medical training, and adheres to a set of predetermined parameters of care.

As an aside, the Ethiopian Athletics Federation (EAF) is a World Athletics-recognized member, representing Ethiopia as the national governing body for all athletic endeavors.[204] EAF was formed on 4 June 1961, and was first noted in the 1960 Olympics as barefooted Abebe Bikila took the gold medal in the Marathon.[204] Bikila repeated in 1964—and the floodgates of Ethiopia as a global powerhouse in long-distance running—were opened. According to its bylaws, EAF seeks to address gaps in athlete's access to physiotherapy and nutrition, as well as education and research programs to upgrade knowledge for coaches and medical staff in sports medicine.[204]

Mengistu explained that, depending on the season, he receives many fall injuries during the rainy season; and conversely, many sports-related injuries (primarily from soccer) during the summer season. He claims to average three to six patients per week.

I first confirm if there is a fracture [via X-rays], then I reduce the fracture. If it is an open fracture, I perform first aid.—*Ayele Mengistu, 75*

> "I first confirm if there is a fracture [via X-rays], then I reduce the fracture. If it is an open fracture, I perform first aid."
>
> *- Ayele Mengistu, 75*

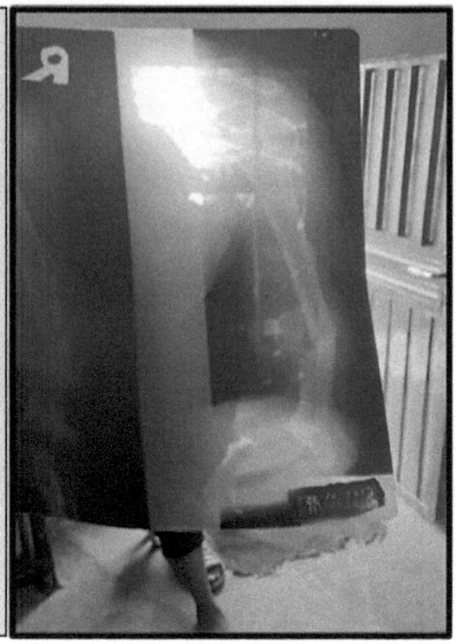

Photo 3.11. Ethiopian bonesetter Mengistu consults hospital X-rays from his fracture patients.

Mengistu stated that when a patient comes to him with a probable fracture, he first confirms "if there is a fracture, then I reduce the fracture." He said if it is an open fracture, he first performs any necessary first aid, or wound care, then he affords the "proper medical treatment" that should be done, including the reduction of the fracture.

At this juncture in this research, it is important for the authors of this book to note that fracture management can be divided into two classifications: nonoperative and operative techniques. The nonoperative approach (used by Mengistu) consists of a closed reduction (if required), followed by a period of immobilization with casting or splinting. Closed reduction is needed if the fracture is significantly displaced or angulated. The goal of fracture reduction is the realignment of the displaced fractured fragments caused by muscle tension or impaction back into the original anatomic relationship. Please note that some fractures are complex and require surgery to place plates, pins, or screws, so the bone(s) can heal properly, other fractures can be successfully reset without surgery (via closed reduction method).

After the patient's fracture reduction, Mengistu states that he "adjusts the muscles to their proper places" using hot water to relieve blood flow and ice for decreasing pain as I deem fit. Wrap done by medical gauze. I usually don't use oral medication, but if need be, Diclofenac or Panadol (NSAIDs). Topical ointments I use are Vaseline infused with black seed, ginger, turmeric [...] or Voltaren (topical NSAID).

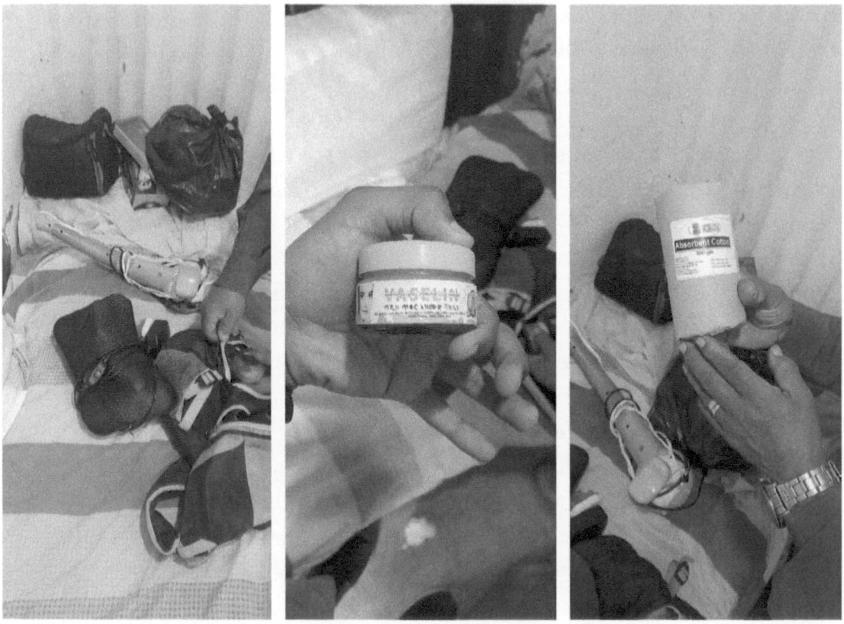

Photo (L to R) 3.12–3.14. Mengistu displays his cache of medical supplies, including muscle stimulator, as well as medical-grade fracture slings, Vaseline, and 100% cotton absorbent gauze roll for wound care.

As a final step, Mengistu explains that he uses "*abish*," known as the 'seed of antiquity' is Ethiopian fenugreek (*Trigonella foenum-graecum*), also spelled '*foenugreek*', is a fragrant herb of the pea family (*Fabaceae*). Globally, *abish* has been reported to have anti-inflammatory and anti-muscular pain properties. In the following published case testimonial, it seems another bonesetter 'prepped' his patient for a procedure via a topical application of *abish*:

> "I wanted to share a little bit of information on the 'medicinal' use of *abish* (fenugreek). In the late 1960's, I saw a traditional physician from Gurage (Eza) using thickly boiled (powdered) *abish* as padding on dislocated shoulder and broken collar bone that he wanted to fix. He left that on for a few days (can't recall exactly how long). He then fixed the socket and the broken collar bone very easily. The patient had dislocated her shoulder and broken the collar bone while riding a horse in Janmeda; Ras Desta Hospital had used their system and left it, but nothing was mended. The traditional bone setter said the fenugreek he applied externally made the bone malleable. His name was Hakim Bayesa, and he had an office in Merkato", said Dr. Tsehai Berhane-Selassie to the Ethiopian Education and Research Network (EEDN).[110pl]

As one of the oldest cultivated plants known to humans, it has been grown in the Nile Valley since 1000 BC. '*Abish*' is grown all over Ethiopia as a popular bread spice, and as a home remedy for digestion/flatulence, leprosy, wound dressing, urinary retention, and joint immobility (vitality of ligaments—oral ingestion).[110,111] '*Foenum-graecum*' means 'hay from Greece, and 'Trigonella' translates to 'little triangle' (mimicking the triangular shape of the small white-yellow flowers) (a.k.a 'goat's horn', or 'cow's horn'), it is used to decreasing pain during a bone-setting procedure by Ethiopian TBS. treatment of boils, cellulitis, tuberculosis, mouth ulcers, and topically for inflammation and myalgia (muscular pain).[111] It has been proposed that saponins and the fiber-rich gum portion of the seeds might contribute to the cholesterol lowering effect, while the galactomannan ingredient may be responsible for the antidiabetic activity.[111] Animal data show that fenugreek inhibits inflammatory swelling,[111] and Fenugreek is also a source of diosgenin, a precursor used in commercial steroid synthesis. Fenugreek grows predominantly in the Mediterranean regions of Africa—Egypt, northern Sudan, Libya, and Tunisia; in northern Africa, it is known by the local Arabic name '*helba*'.[111]

IN THEIR OWN WORDS: Adwoa Kuma, 90, and Peter Dwamena, 50—Bonesetter & Apprentice, Ghana

The third and fourth bonesetters that were interviewed were a duo of a 90-year-old elderly man and his younger 50-year-old apprentice, Adwoa Kuma and Peter Dwamena (Akumsa Dumase, Ghana). Neither Kuma nor Dwamena received any formal institutionalized education, however Dwamena said he has seen what an X-rays looks like. Kuma and Dwamena represent an almost five-generation familial bone-setting business. Kuam's daughter works as a bonesetter in a nearby village and creates all of the treatment powders the three utilize for minor injuries.

> "It's the medicine
> that's powerful.
> It's the type of plant or
> tree-
> the leaves, bark, or
> roots -
> that does the work."
>
> *-Adwoa Kuma, go*

The pair claim to serve approximately 100 patients per year. "It's the medicine that's powerful. It's the type of plant or tree—the leaves, bark, or roots—that does the work." "It's a gift, a spiritual blessing, the bonesetter must give to the person so they can have the power to heal the bones. The spiritual blessing is necessary, and once you are in the family and working as a bonesetter, you can get the ceremonial rites."

According to the pair of bonesetters, several plants they utilize include Odom (*Milicia regia*), which is a tree that grows in a belt that extends from Zanzibar on the east coast of Africa to Gambia on the west coast.[112] The bark is used by Kuma Dwamena for closed fractures; they also have their patients ingest the ground bark. Another very well-known plant the pair uses is the "Pawpaw", a tropical fruit (also known as a type of papaya), with a small deciduous tree that produces large yellowish-green fruit. The fruit has long been believed to contain healthful properties that boost digestion and immunity, and aid in diabetes and arthritis control.[112] Ghana papaya is cultivated on a large scale in the regions of greater Accra, central, eastern and Volta.[112] Kuma and Dwamena used the Pawpaw leaves for wounds and open fractures.

Other Ghanaian roots, leaves, bark, flowers, and fruits used by the bonesetters in traditional medicines include (but are not limited to): Whitei (*Mondia Whitei*), or white's ginger root, is an endangered, perennial, woody and resilient climbing plant that grows from a tuberous root. Researchers have tested various extracts for aphrodisiac, antidepressant, anti-inflammatory, antibacterial, and antiepileptic activities, however the most promising studies seem to focus primarily to aphrodisiac activity efficacy.[113] Kuma and Dwamena used the Whitei root for open fracture care. The last ingredient Kuma and Dwamena mention using for fracture care is '*Efom Wisa*'—a type of West African black pepper. *Efom wisa* (also known as 'Grains of Paradise', Alligator Pepper, Guinea Pepper) and is from the ginger family *Zingiberaceae*. Kuma and Dwamena use *Wisa* in the patient's ingested drink mix. However, in one Nigerian study conducted on rats, researchers concluded that the ingestion of large quantities of Alligator pepper (*zingiberaceae aframomum melegueta*) "poses a health risk to women in their first trimester of pregnancy".[114p163]

IN THEIR OWN WORDS: Portia Rutendo Machokoto, 69, Bonesetter, Zimbabwe

Our only female bonesetter interview came from the Midlands Province (Gokwe Nembudziya), in Zimbabwe. Portia Rutendo Machokoto (see Photo 3.15).

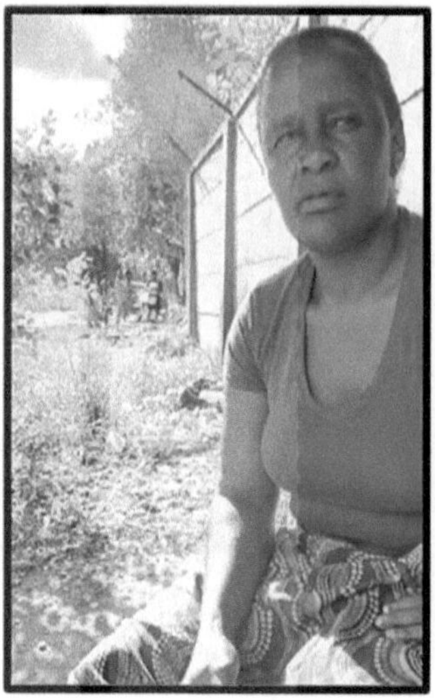

"I was called by the ancestors to heal... Unfortunately, a lot of people now go to the hospital for healing."

- Portia Rutendo Machokoto, 69

Photo 3.15. A local bonesetter, explained that she had no official training, as she "was called by the ancestors". She refused to give us more information on how she was bequeathed her role, as it is not allowed by her ancestors to tell their secrets. She then referred us to Zimbabwe National Traditional Healers Association for more information on how traditional healers receive their calling. She concluded by stating that she is a merely a "vessel of her ancestors" and she works "as they please [at their pleasure]".

She said that in her area the nearest hospital is about 20 kilometers (approximately 12.5 miles) away, and only those with oxcarts can travel easily but the majority of the community is very poor, therefore they seek assistance from traditional healers like her. Portia does not rely on X-rays or any process(es) of Western medicine; instead, she employs only her hands, her eyes, and the 'divine guidance' from her ancestors. During our interview, there was problem with taking any photographs. The bonesetter explained that in order to show what she does, we needed to sacrifice a goat in order to appease the ancestors. Therefore, if we wanted 'evidence' of the healing, Portia said via translator, we had to "enter the rituals to experience her at work."

According to Portia, the number of patients she treats "depends on the ancestors and those who need divine healing," she said, "The world needs healing and it's up to us [them] to heal it." According to the interviewers' observations, the consensus was that she averages up to three clients per month, helping people with different bone needs. She said that the number is lower than it was in back in the 1990s. She attributes this decrease mainly "because of many religions that caused the eradication of ancestral culture."

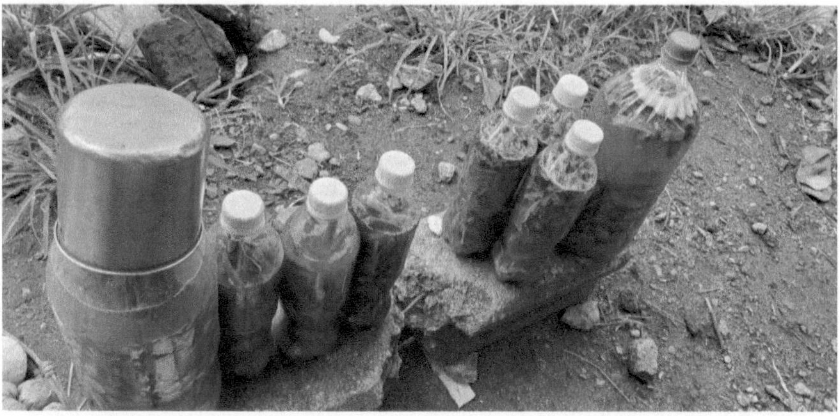

Photo 3.16. Portia explained the green leaves of the *Anesellia* (*Ansellia Africana*) are used right when a patient first arrives to drink "so that the germs or infection will come out", much like an antibiotic. When it's dry, they mix it in water for a week (or so), and then give to the patient to drink, she said it helps to stop the pain and also "helps the bones to be strong." She also uses the *Warburgia salutaris*, also known as Muranga (Shona), or the Pepper-bark tree (English). This *Warburgia* plant she uproots – stem and the roots. It is dried and ground into a powder. It is applied on the fracture (on the bone) and then she bandages the wound with cloth. She said after every week the patient he/she has to come back for dressing the wound till it closes.

Yes, she stated, she can help those with 'open wounds' (open fractures), as she uses her herbs to stop the bleeding. She also uses a medicinal tree bark to close the wound just like a bandage. Unfortunately, she said sadly, a lot of people now rely on Western medicine hospital. She did mention that she has not received an open wound bone fracture in more than two years. The cost for her treatment? Portia smiles and says it depended on the type of bone break. People pay "a hen, goat, or sheep" depending on how much they can afford, she said. Sometimes I do it for free if the ancestors tell me so. As for money, I accept what is given with a willing heart. The issue of money can cause problems sometimes, she clarified, so I don't charge.

IN THEIR OWN WORDS: Philip Chimoya, 67, Bonesetter, Zimbabwe

Philip, a local bonesetter, works in the Masvingo Province in Zimbabwe. He explained he received no professional healthcare training, as his healing powers come from "a call from the ancestors". Admittedly, he said he has sporadically attended community workshops for traditional healers offered by the Zimbabwe National Traditional Healers Association (ZINATHA).[115] Sometimes ZINATHA refers patients who have bone fractures to him—however only if the patients trust traditional medicine. We were refused permission to enter his 'healing room' as it is not open for public viewing. Specifically, outsiders that wish to enter must first "ask the ancestors" through various exercises and/or invocations of supernatural powers, such as brewing beer and slaughtering a goat. Philip, born in January of 1956, was also adamant that if outsiders wished to witness his 'healing processes', he would (again) first need to gain "permission from the ancestors" as "no phones or cameras are allowed" during the healing process as it is a traditional process that does not allow new technologies to be present.

According to Philip (see Photo 3.17 below), his local Masvingo province has the "largest number of patients who use traditional medication". We estimated that he treats approximately seven clients per month, each with varying issues, such as open fracture, closed fracture, back pain, joint pain, etc. Philip also explained that his current number of patients has steadily decreased, as many young(er) Zimbabweans are now turning to Western hospitals and medications.

"Healing is not free. It is not allowed to pay with money. You must pay with sheep, goats, cattle or hens."

- Philip Chimoya, 67

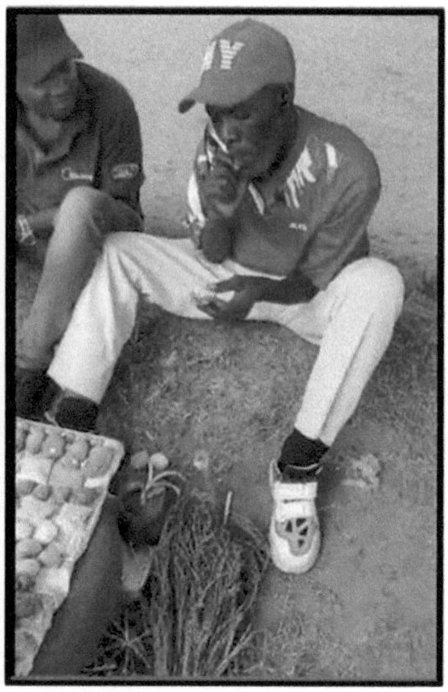

Photo 3.17. Male Zimbabwean bonesetter, Philip.

Philip's clients who visit him with bone problems have closed and open bone fractures. He explains that in his area the nearest hospital is about 50 kilometers away, and only those who have transport can travel there easily. So, that is why most of the community members come and seek help from him and other traditional healers, as they cannot afford transport fares and the hospital bills. He does not use X-ray or any Western medicine, instead he uses his spiritual guidance granted to him from the ancestors.

When asked how much he charges for his TBS fees, he said that it all depends on how big the wound is or the fracture. Most patients pay him with hens, goats, or sheep. But this all depends on how much the patient and their family can afford. He did mention that the treatment is not free and it is not allowed to pay with [cash] money, so payment must be made in-kind, in the form of livestock, such as cattle, goats and hens.

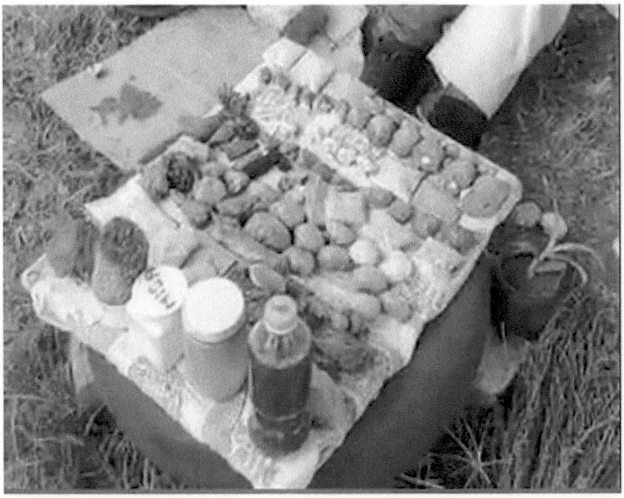

Photo 3.18. Philip's 'medical bag', laid out with oral remedies and ointments, etc.

As for his utilization of herbal medicines, Philip said he uses the *Dicoma anomala* plant 'Chifumuro' or 'Fever bush' on open wounds. He gives it to the patient to use on a daily basis until the fracture is dry. He places roots of the *Dicoma anomala* plant in warm water, then uses the leftover water to wash the fracture daily. As for the well-known African aloe vera plant, he explained to us that there are many different types of aloe vera plant. The particular type he utilizes is only the one "which grows in-between rocks." He extracts the 'juice' from the leaves, then applies it directly on the fracture. He claims that the aloe vera gel "kills all the germs" and any "viruses on the wound." He also uproots (stem and roots) of the *Warburgia salutaris* plant. He dries it out, grinds it into a powder and then applies it on the fractured bones directly. After the medical plant remedies, he then bandages the patient's broken bones. The patient must come back to him on a weekly basis for his application of a fresh bandage dressing.

Like other African bonesetters and healers, Philip also utilizes the Leopard orchid, or *Ansellia africana*. Philip explained that "uproots the entire plant"—an endangered species of orchid which is severely threatened and declining due to over-collecting for commercial and medicinal use.[112] He then grinds it and allows it dry in the sun. He puts the powder in a bottle with water, instructing the patient to drink it daily over the next 7–14 days. Philip reported that this remedy "helps the bones to be strong." Unfortunately, Philip refused to allow us to meet any of his prior patients. He claimed that his association (which is ZINATHA)[115] does not allow them, if we wanted to interview the patients we have to go and get the letter from them which will grant us access to patients in the community.

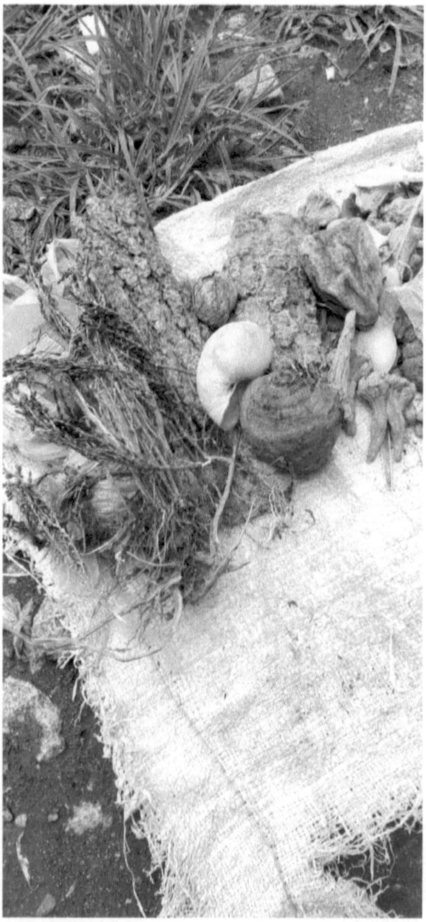

Photos 3.19. The Zimbabwean bonesetter's mixture of shells, roots, bark, leaves and roots that will make up a remedy.

IN THEIR OWN WORDS: Moses, 21, Former TBS Patient, Ghana

The authors met with one of Daniel's former patients, Moses, a 21-year-old man. Moses explained that six months ago, he had an accident on his motorbike. He said due to a (closed) fractured femur (thighbone) and open fractures of his tibia (shinbone) and fibula; he sought medical care at Wenchi Hospital in the city of Wenchi. After two months and a 7,500-cedi (approx. $1,286 USD) hospital bill, Moses had his splinting removed. With two nurses and one doctor in his hospital room, Moses attempted to walk for the first time since his motorbike accident. Unaided and unsteady—Moses fell forcefully to the hard cement floor, reinjuring his leg. After the incident, he left Wenchi Hospital against medical advice (AMA). Moses' sister entreated him to travel 43 miles to undergo Daniel's traditional bone-setting care.

Now, after six weeks of Daniel's treatment, Moses said he "feels stronger" and can walk better. However, Daniel must rely on the use of a crutch, his leg is deformed and his gait is permanently impaired as the injured leg has shortened due to an improper healing and malalignment of bones. Western evidence-based scientific research has shown that a broken leg bone can lead to a 'limb length discrepancy' if the leg heals in an overlapped or shortened position, if the skin and muscle tissue around the bone were severely injured and exposed (as occurs in a high-energy trauma open fracture), or if there is a 'malunion' or 'nonunion' of the leg due to a lack of adequate stability, blood flow, or both, according to Admasu.

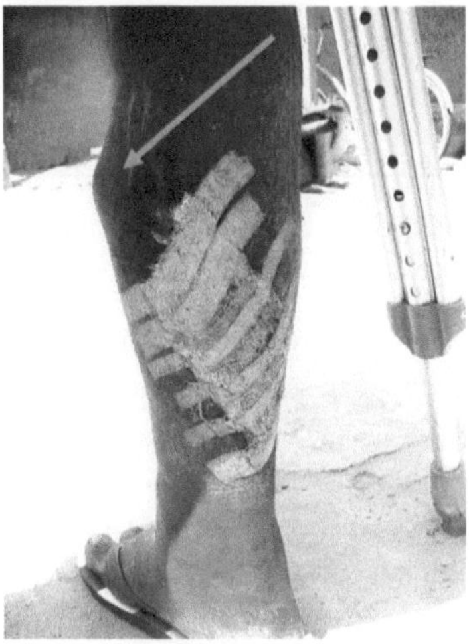

Photo 3.20. Photo showing post-TBS patient Moses, 21, with deformity and impaired gait.

IN THEIR OWN WORDS: James, 27, Current TBS Patient, Ghana

Another one of Daniel's former patients, James, age 30, sought the bonesetter's help after falling off of a roof while performing some construction work some 5 years ago. Right after his fall, James went to Ahmadiyya Muslim Hospital in Techiman. The staff there told him he did not need an X-rays, as he had a 'sore inside the bone'. While they did offer James some ointment for his back and free pain medication, he complained that none of what the Ahmadiyya staff offered him helped ease his acute back pain.

Therefore, every three days, James travels 27 miles to have Daniel apply his '*dufa*' and massage his back with hot water. Upon physical inspection of James' torso, a rash was painfully evident: "The power of the medicine will at times make a rash," James explained.

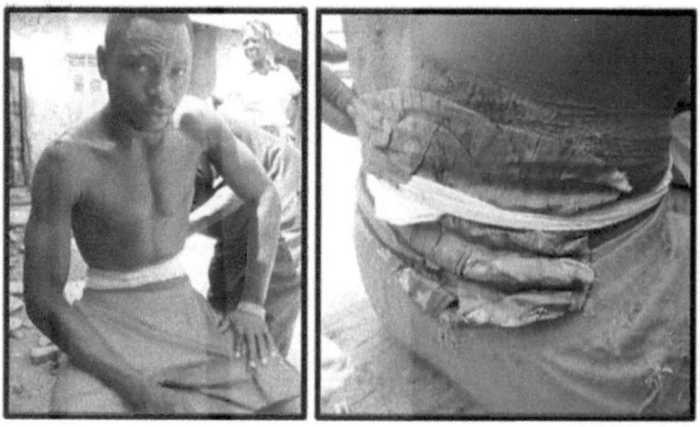

"The power of the medicine will at times make a rash."

-Robert Fosu Appiah, 56

Photo 3.21–3.22. (L) James showing his tightly bandaged back. (R) James has Daniel apply paste and bandages every three days.

IN THEIR OWN WORDS: Hardlife Mandishona, 27, Former TBS Patient, Zimbabwe

Six months ago, twenty-seven-year-old Hardlife (who refused to be photographed) was involved in an oxcart accident. His cart hit a ditch and the axle was broken. This caused the oxcart to turn upside down. He was in a lot of pain, and then found he couldn't move his right leg well. Hardlife, however, realized that his right leg was broken, even though he had a closed fracture. Since the hospital was too far, he was rushed to Portia Machokoto where he was given herbs to drink and some medical poultices to apply on the injured leg. In less than half of one year, Hardlife now is able to walk with the assistance of a cane.

IN THEIR OWN WORDS: Tobaiwanenhamo Hamutyinei, 49, Current TBS Patient, Zimbabwe

Late at night in December of 2022, Mr. Hamutyinei (who refused to be photographed) fell and broke his arm on his way out of a local *shebeen*. A '*shebeen*' is an informal alcohol outlet, or an unlicensed establishment (or private house) selling alcohol. That same night, he was rushed to the bonesetter, Portia Machokoto, and was given herbs to drink and poultices to apply directly on the (closed) fracture. He explained that he does "not trust Western medicine" because it "causes other diseases" and had "bad side effects," which is why he only utilizes traditional medicine. One month later, he is still under the bonesetter's care and actively "healing", the patient stated.

Medically Authenticated Post-TBS Case #1—Tesfaye

Tesfaye (a fictitious name) is 27 years old. Two weeks before his visit to the hospital, he was in a road traffic accident on his way to work from his hometown. He remembers experiencing severe pain in his left knee and leg, which he was unable to move. He was then taken to a clinic near the site of the accident and was referred to the city for specialist care. But once his family arrived at the clinic (after receiving a phone call that he was at clinic), everything changed. His brothers, father, and other family members insisted that he should go to a traditional bonesetter rather than traveling many kilometers to the city's specialized hospital. Tesfaye also believed that the treatment by the bonesetter would be very good—if not better than that offered at the public university hospital in Gondar. The family members exhaustively also enumerated and discussed the various people that they knew who had been (somewhat successfully) treated by this specific bonesetter.

Once at the bonesetter, Tesfay's acutely injured limb was aggressively kneaded and manipulated by the TBS—despite his cries due to the significant pain. The bonesetter told him that he had a knee dislocation, and that he had successfully "put it back in place." Despite the inordinate amount of pain, Tesfaye held on to hope for a full and timely recovery. However, as the days passed, his leg began to feel cold and numb, with his skin darkened to a sickly looking pitch-black color. It was only then that Tesfaye decided to return to the clinic. Once there, he was, yet again, referred to the city's large urban hospital. This time, though, he followed the staff's accurate healthcare advice and visited the specialized hospital.

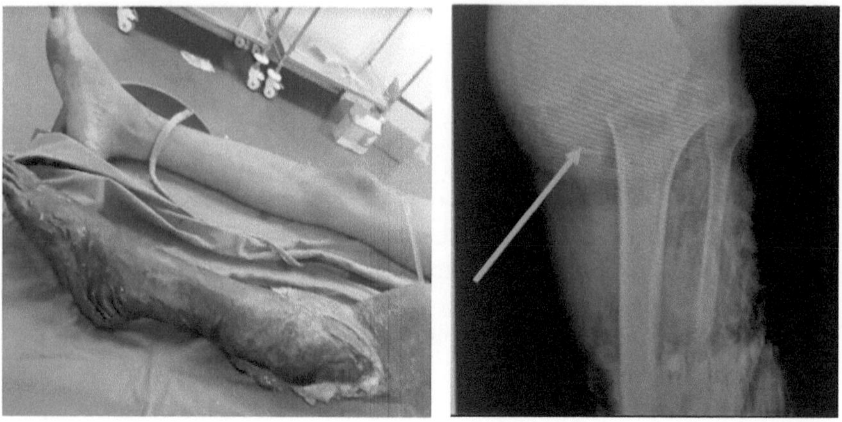

Photo 3.23–3.24. (L) An unreduced knee fracture and dislocation from a road traffic accident, treated by a traditional Ethiopian bonesetter. (R) X-rays confirming dislocation and fracture.

The doctor's noted that at presentation, the patient's lower extremity had a gross visible deformity. The leg was dark, cold, and had no sensation, pulse, pain, or movement. Hospital X-rays confirmed posterior knee dislocation, and a Doppler exam showed an absence of peripheral blood flow starting at the popliteal fossa (where a thrombus was blocking the artery). With this diagnosis, and due to the patient's late presentation of the blood clot, an above-knee amputation was immediately advised.

At the news of a possible amputation of his leg, Tesfaye began crying uncontrollably. He was in a state of disbelief that it was medically necessary from him to undergo a surgical amputation. His family members were furious at the mere suggestion of a limb amputation. Tesfaye was given time to consider his options, as the surgical intervention was going to be a life-altering one. He knew that whether he decided to amputate—or refuse the amputation—both were ending his life (and future livelihood in rural Ethiopia) as he knew it. It took Tesfaye more than 18 hours to decide. He finally agreed to the procedure. He gave consent and an above-knee amputation was performed. In subsequent days, his amputation stump was healing well, however, Tesfaye was depressed and while recuperating in the hospital's Orthopedic ward, he ate sparingly, slept poorly, and spoke very little to the surrounding patients, staff, and visiting family members.

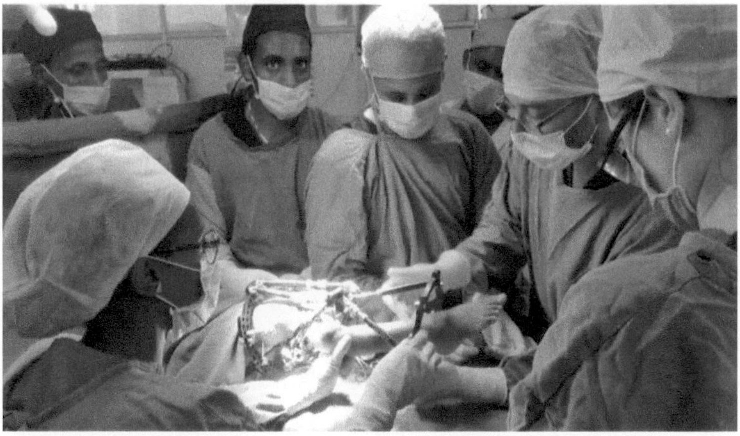

Photo 3.25. Dr. Ananya Admasu (on right foreground) during a modern-day pediatric orthopedic surgery in progress in 2023 at University of Gondar's Comprehensive Hospital in Gondar, Ethiopia.

Medically Authenticated Post-TBS Case #2—Solomon

Solomon, a 25-year-old farmer, got into a quarrel with his family members over a land dispute. At the end of the quarrel, he had sustained a bullet injury from an AK-47. He was in pain and bleeding. He went to a traditional bonesetter nearby who dressed the wound with a mixture of leaves and other (undisclosed) ingredients and wrapped it in cloth bandages. Solomon went back home but was unable to walk or perform his daily work functions. Despite becoming bedbound, Solomon continued visiting the bonesetter for periodic treatment sessions.

As time progressed, he noticed that his toes had started to darken, and there was a foul-smelling discharge coming from his wound. He then decided to visit a nearby clinic, whose staff referred him to a specialized regional hospital. When he presented to the specialized hospital, he already had darkened toes, the skin over his leg was sloughed, and there was pus draining from a mid-leg wound (about 3 cm × 4 cm posteriorly), a pinpoint exit wound (lateral distal leg), and distal pulses were not palpable. The X-rays showed no fracture present; however, a Doppler reading showed the tibialis posterior was transected high in the leg. Both an erythrocyte sedimentation rate (ESR) and white blood cell test were elevated, revealing inflammatory activity.

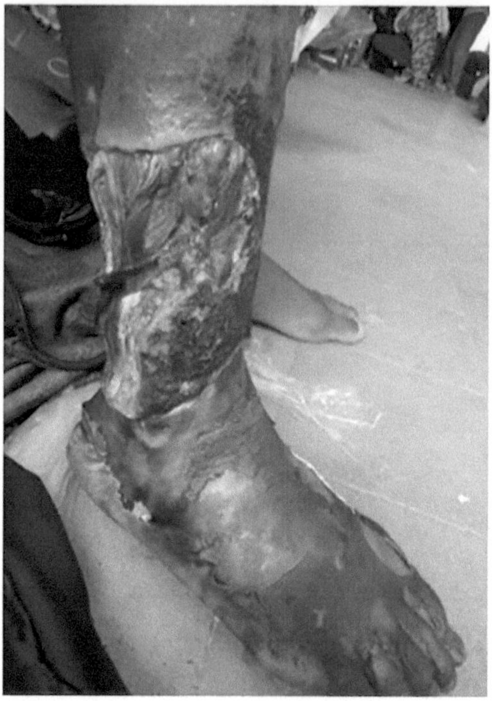

Photo 3.26. Wet gangrene after an AK-47 gunshot wound to the foot in Ethiopia. Patient was treated by traditional bonesetter. At hospital presentation, distal pulses were not palpable, and a Doppler reading showed the tibialis posterior was transected high in the leg.

Solomon was informed of his test results, and the diagnosis of wet gangrene was disclosed to his family. It was crucial that the spread of infection systemically be avoided by removing the source of the infection; therefore, amputation at a higher level (to make sure of a clean margin) was advised. Solomon, like so many other pre-amputation patients, refused the procedure.

After he was given time to think, he placed a condition that he would only agree to the amputation if it was done at the level of the injury and no higher. He was advised about all the possible risks of sepsis, septic shock, and the mortality associated with his decision. However, Solomon was not willing to reconsider. The hospital team acquiesced to some of the patient's terms and explained that a secondary operation may be needed if the infection was not controlled, and/or intraoperatively if the remaining tissue looked infected. The amputation was performed at the hospital successfully and the patient had a full recovery.

Medically Authenticated Post-TBS Case # 3—Sefiw

Sefiw, a 15-year-old male from Chilga, Ethiopia, presented to the hospital with an injury from a fall, a trauma that took place one week prior to his arrival. His parents had previously taken him to a local traditional bonesetter. The bonesetter painfully manipulated and aggressively massaged his arm with butter. The TBS then tightly wrapped the fracture with bamboo sticks and strips of cloth below his elbow. Sefiw explained that he was in severe pain, but he was told that a fracture is 'expected to hurt' until it is fully healed. His growing discomfort was both normalized and marginalized by the TBS and his family. Despite the bonesetter's treatment, Sefiw was having great difficulty moving his fingers and the (uncovered) visible parts of his hand remained extremely swollen. Finally, after one week, the boy's uncle decided to bring him to a specialized Western medical hospital in Gondar.

At presentation, there was swelling both in the hand and the forearm with gross deformity around the wrist. He had some movement in his fingers, but it was difficult and painful. The X-rays showed a distal radial

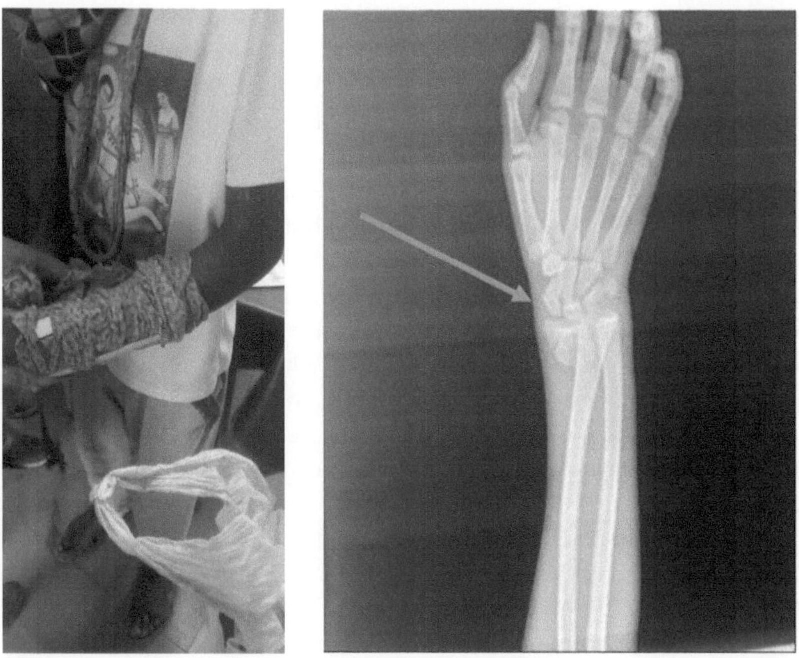

Photo 3.27–3.28. (L) Parents allow their son's fracture to be treated by traditional bonesetter – however, an uncle intervened and brought child to a medical hospital in order to receive appropriate fracture-reduction treatment and a modern splint. (R) X-rays confirming fracture.

extra-articular fracture with shortening and dorsal angulations. He and his uncle were advised to allow an attempt a closed reduction by the orthopedic staff. However, one of the boy's parents had to be present to sign a consent for the minor. So, the parents were phoned and his father traveled in to the hospital the following day. The closed reduction procedure was successful in realigning the fracture, and a proper radial gutter splint was applied. Upon the boy's discharge from the hospital, PT of the hand, elbow, and shoulder were prescribed to assist in full restorative movement and limb function.

Medically Authenticated Post-TBS Case #4—Daniel

Twelve-year-old Daniel was outside looking after the family's cattle and while he was trying to herd them back to safety, he suddenly fell off a cliff. He fell in the afternoon and was not discovered until late evening—hours later when his father and uncles went to search for him. He was in agonizing pain when they found him. They immediately took him to a nearby bonesetter. The bonesetter massaged his fracture—at which point Daniel lost consciousness from the pain. The bonesetters' massage and manipulation were followed by the bandaging of the boy's forearm with sticks and strips of cloth.

Daniel said he experienced excruciating pain over the next few weeks. His family were told repeatedly that the child's discomfort "is normal, that's how his body is healing" by the bonesetter. They trusted him and did their best to comfort the boy's distress. However, as the days went by, he had a foul-smelling 'fluid' oozing out of the bandages and he was finding it hard to move his fingers. His father decided to bring him to the large public hospital in Gondar. After three weeks, he had already developed wet gangrene of the forearm. Wet gangrene occurs when bacteria invade the tissue, making the area swell, drain fluid, and reek. Sadly, the family was informed about the poor prognosis, and the only feasible solution—amputation. But his father refused to consider the concept even remotely. The parents and family were warned of the possibilities of sepsis (the body's extreme response to an infection; a life-threatening medical emergency) and septic shock (also a life-threatening condition that happens when your blood pressure drops to a dangerously low level after an infection), conditions which would occur if the infection remained untreated. However, the father insisted that he would not allow the child to lose his arm, despite doctor's recommendations.

After the doctor's prognosis, the father returned to his village and, again, sought the counsel and assistance of the bonesetter. Nevertheless, one week later, Daniel, his father, and his uncles were back at the emergency department of the hospital in Gondar. Unfortunately, by now, the boy's forearm was necrotic (or the death of tissue due to no blood flow; an

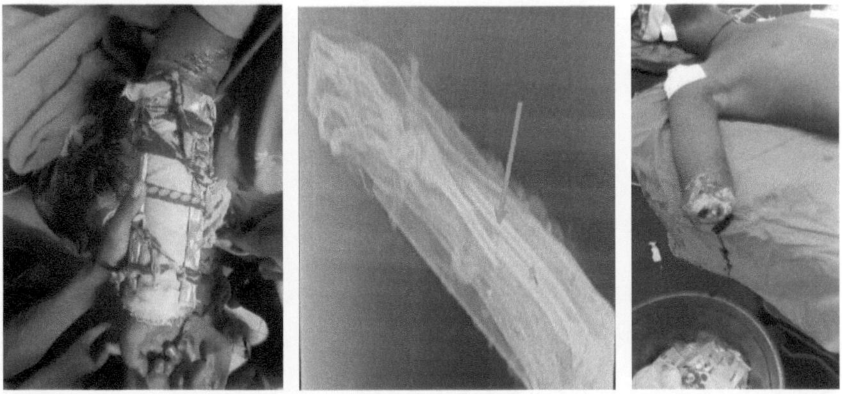

Photo 3.29–3.31. (L to R) The patient's forearm at presentation in the ED. (Middle) X-rays showing the closed fracture, a lack of reduction of the fracture, and the ensuing infection and necrotic tissues. (R) This is how the post-trans-humeral-amputation 'open site' was left to heal.

irreversible condition) below the elbow, and the child was extremely ill from the infection. After evaluation and initial stabilization, the father begged the surgeons to 'spare as much limb' as possible. Daniel was taken to the operating theater that same night and a trans-humeral amputation was performed. Subsequently, he had a prolonged hospital stay due to his open post-operative stump (note: an open site, where the incision is not sewn or stapled closed, allows staff to monitor and remove any infected tissue that might have been left behind).

Medically Authenticated Post-TBS Case #5—Ermias

Ermias is a ninth grader who was playing soccer with his friends at school when he fell abruptly and awkwardly on his left arm. He was in a great deal of pain and unable to move his left arm. The school called his parents and told them to take him to the hospital; however, they chose to take him to a local bonesetter in their rural town instead. Their assumption was that since he was young, he probably had a dislocation (not a fracture), and the simple injury could be treated with the limited intervention of a bonesetter. The bonesetter advised Ermias to have daily massages of melted butter on the injured site every day until the dislocation 'popped' back into place. Ermias said he hated every moment of the bonesetter's treatment, and the pain and swelling were increasing daily—rather than decreasing. After a week, the teenager abruptly refused to go to the bonesetter for the painful machinations.

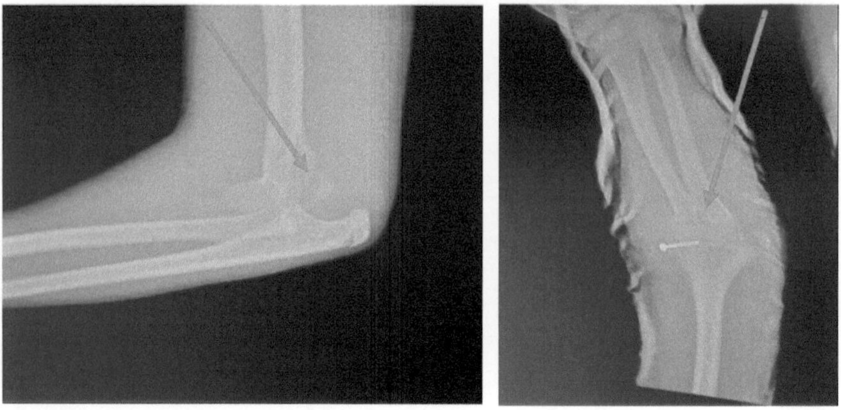

Photo 3.32–3.33. (L) One-week post-TBS pre-op fracture dislocation. (R) Surgical intervention.

However, his parents did convince him that he should at least visit the hospital he, and he readily agreed. He was taken to the hospital one week after his injury. He was diagnosed with a fracture dislocation of the left elbow. They were advised that the staff would make an attempt of a closed reduction. Nonetheless, there was a possibility of failure, and then only a surgical reduction would be possible. Unfortunately, due to the extensive bony and soft tissue injury involved, the nonsurgical closed reduction failed, so Ermias underwent a successful surgical intervention. After two days in the hospital, he was discharged.

Medically Authenticated Post-TBS Case #6—UUE (Nigeria)

Without a doubt, the most egregious case study we have reviewed on bonesetter intervention is found through Abang et al. (2022) in Nigeria.[116] This particular aforementioned case study bears mention in that six traumatologists and surgeons from the Department of Orthopedics and Traumatology at the University of Calabar, Nigeria, verified the patient outcome via X-rays, photos, and laboratory testing—and sent out a global warning that there is a marked increase of 'quacks' who now 'dabble' in complex orthopedic surgeries. Case in point: A traditional bonesetter in collaboration with "some health workers (quacks who were community health extension workers) engaged in performing an open reduction and internal fixation for a femoral fracture."[116p21] The six doctors said they published this case study to "illustrate the extent of malpractices by traditional bonesetters" who are now being actively assisted by untrained health workers—who have at some time, perhaps, assisted or watched orthopedic procedures in an operating room.[116p21]

According to the study, a 28-year-old male student was in a motorcycle accident and when he regained consciousness, he was receiving IV fluids and his thigh was bandaged. After one week, the traditional bonesetter and the community health worker began the complex surgery that the young student had agreed to, most willingly. Post operatively, the student suffered from severe wound infections, was unable to walk, and fell—whereby the bonesetter's blunt, unsterile metal construction strip with holes (manufactured for use in wood) painfully burst through the skin, several screws fell out of the wound site, and a pus-filled discharge oozed out of the thigh.[116]

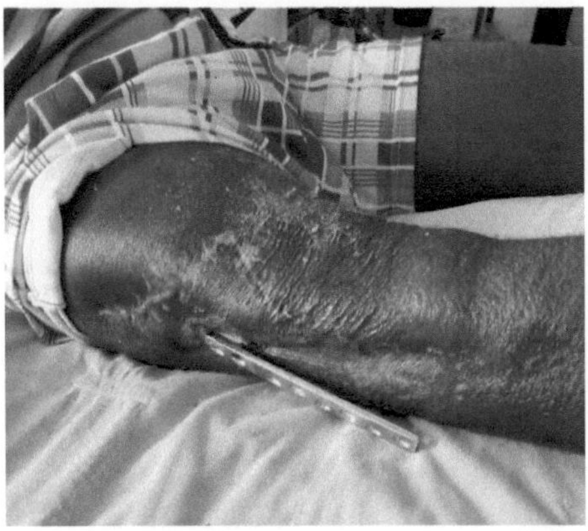

Photo 3.34. The exposed implant on the right femur. Photo copyright Dr. Innocent Abang, 2022.

Upon a medical inspection, the doctors reported: a limb length discrepancy (LLD) of 12 cm; a reduced range of motion across the hip and knee; *Staphylococcus aureus* and *Pseudomonas aeriginosa* infections; loosening of plate and screws; and a bone loss in proximal femur at fracture site (with gap of 4 cm), so a diagnosis of "infected atrophic non-union with bone loss of proximal right femur" with exposed metal plate was delivered.[116p23] See Photo 3.34. Unbelievably, this toxic combination of untrained health workers collaborating with TBS is "gradually emerging" and "features of quackery are often demonstrated in their injudicious massages, poor diagnosis and misplaced treatment resulting in very unpleasant complications like nonunion, malunion, delayed union, sometimes outright gangrene of the limb" (due to vascular compromise), according to the case study physicians.[116p23] This is a preposterous open-and-shut case of intentional malpractice (not iatrogenic injury, which is caused unintentionally) by a reckless bonesetter, and breaks the oldest and most sanctioned rule of medical ethics: *primum non nocere*, or above all, do no harm.

In conclusion, while these handful of traditional bonesetters, their patients, and their orthopedic surgeons may not represent the myriads of possible patient outcomes, the medically authenticated cases do serve to illustrate how aggressive bonesetter manipulations of fracture sites and soft tissues, mismanagement of traction, splinting, and unsterile, invasive implants, and patient referral delays play an undeniably detrimental role in patient outcomes. That being said, some positive traditional healings do occur, and have occurred for millennia, and there is, incontrovertibly, enormous value to the safe and judicious use of all-natural flora and fauna products for healing a variety of non-acute wounds, toothaches, diarrhea, some skin rashes, headaches, constipation, bodily pains, etc.. We will now, in our subsequent chapter, investigate the global importance of scientifically credible, robust ethnopharmacological inquiry.

Chapter 4

PHYTOCHEMISTRY, PHARMACOGNOSY, AND ETHNOBOTANICS

To date, some 40,000–70,000 plant species have been screened for their ethnopharmacological uses, and of the 122 drugs derived from medicinal plants which are in use worldwide, 80% can be traced back to their ethnomedicinal uses.[117] As Ciddi Veeresham (2012) noted in his *Journal of Advanced Technology and Research* article: "Natural Products Derived from Plants as a Source of Drugs," nature furnishes our integral bioactive components:

> Nature, the master of craftsman of molecules created almost an inexhaustible array of molecular entities. It stands as an infinite resource for drug development, novel chemotypes and pharmacophores, and scaffolds for amplification into efficacious drugs for a multitude of disease indications and other valuable bioactive agents. Since time immemorial, natural products have been the backbone of traditional system of healing throughout the globe and have also been an integral part of history and culture. Although the use of bioactive natural products as herbal drug preparations dates back hundreds, even thousands, of years ago, their application as isolated and characterized compounds to modern drug discovery and development started only in the 19th century [...] Until recently, plants were an important source of novel pharmacologically active compounds with many blockbuster drugs being derived directly or indirectly from plants. Despite the current preoccupation with synthetic chemistry as a vehicle to discover and manufacture drugs—the contribution of plants to disease treatment and prevention is still enormous. Even at the dawn of 21st century, 11% of the 252 drugs considered as basic and essential by the WHO were exclusively of flowering plant origin.[118p200]

What we found insightful in Nkongmeneck et al.'s (2011) study was that many 'pharmacologically interesting medicinal plant species' in use around the world are employed in more than one community (and usually in more than one country) for multiple uses.[24] We view this as a postulation that global healers have a spot-on awareness of (at least some) of the beneficial phytochemical properties of these items, and have used them successfully to provide remedies for a variety of illnesses. But, among the many challenges facing local pharmaceutical production, like the decentralization of some African health care systems, the underutilization of some rural facilities, and the over-dependance on untested, imported medications.

Precursors to Drugs: Plants and Non-synthetics

Medicinal plants have been utilized (via various extraction methods) in traditional healthcare systems since prehistoric times—and it can be argued—the single-most important healthcare resource for the vast majority of the world's population. Innumerable peer-reviewed studies support the folkloric, or traditional, use of natural plant extracts, fruits, leaves, roots, flowers, and tree bark have, without question, demonstrated potent anti-plasmodial, anti-diabetic, antimicrobial, antifungal, and other effects under Good Laboratory Practices (GLP)—documentation, sampling, testing, ongoing stability program, technical transfer of testing methods—and properly realized phytochemical screenings.

Pharmacognosy is the study of medicines or crude drugs produced from bioactive natural agents such as plants, microbes, and animals. It includes analysis of their biological, chemical, biochemical, and physical properties. At its physiological core, it may well be that the human body assimilates plant-derived medical substances, as they contain easy-to-tolerate non-synthetic elements. Pharmacognosy is generally considered the "oldest brand of pharmacy"[119p1] with an excavated 5,000-year-old Sumerian clay tablet detailing 12 recipes of remedies using poppy and mandrake plants. According to Fields, approximately 25% of prescription medicines in the United States are believed to have an active ingredient from a natural source; in developing countries about 80% of residents rely on traditional medicines made from plants.[119] A plant's active ingredient can be anywhere in its physical structure (such as petal, root, leaf, or stem). In its (unmodified) natural form, it may be inert (chemically inactive), therefore a (or any combinations of) chemical processing, compounding, or chemical reaction(s) may be needed to obtain it in its active form.

One cannot ignore the absence of "institutional support for production and dissemination of key species for cultivation; the low prices paid for traditional medicinal plants by herbal medicine traders and urban herbalists; lack of appropriate technology for post-harvest and pre-processing purposes adapted productively [...] insufficient documentation and scientific experimentation for verification [...] [as well as] lack of preservation of medicinal extracts for extended shelf life," according to Fokunang et al.[3p286] There is no doubt that these developments in understanding traditional medicine were important developments in medical history—as such a valorization comes with systemic scientific processes to create monitoring systems, fund research, record treatment methodologies, and develop patient-safe folk medicine remedies. No one can claim that this would produce an 'all-African approach', instead it would serve to enhance the global standing of traditional medicine's undeniable contribution to public health.

Fields also explained that plants are the source of many active ingredients used for medicinal purposes, some examples include (but are not limited to) the following: salicylic acid; caffeine; *Fusarium pallidoroseum* (the origin of apicidin, a fungal metabolite presenting antiprotozoal activity in vitro that may counter malaria factor); *Plasmodium berghei*; *Taxus Baccata*, or yew tree (used to extract Baccatin III, which is important in the production of some antineoplastic, anticancer, drugs); *Hericium erinaceus*, or lion's mane mushroom (a fungus that shows some evidence of improving nerve and cognitive function); *Catharanthus roseus*, or the Madagascar periwinkle (source of 70+ indole alkaloids, suppressing the metaphase of cellular mitosis—the origin of medicines for childhood leukemia and Hodgkin's disease(s); *Aloe marlothii*, or mountain aloe (used in treatment for intestinal parasites; and *Rumex acetosella*, or the common sorrel (shows diuretic properties and is used as an approach for sinusitis and bronchitis.[119]

Other common household spices, like Tumeric (*Curcuma longa*) [Family: Zingiberaceae], have been studied and sold in American groceries for decades not only for their food flavoring, but also their documented health advantages. As one of the most studied spices in the world, turmeric, is notable in its bioavailability (absorption), recognized safety, and wide breadth of potential benefits.[254] For instance, one 2020 study (by Sharifi-Rad et al.) reported that *Curcuma* (turmeric's biologically active compound) held anti-inflammatory, anticancer, antidiabetic, antidiarrheal, antimicrobial, antiviral, and antioxidant properties.[120]

In our own survey of available studies, we were fascinated by Coda Toafode et al.'s (2022) ethnomedicinal information on plants used for the treatment of bone fractures in the Northern Region of the Republic of Benin, whereby the researchers offer a detailed study of wild plants used by 60 traditional healers for bone fractures.[121] The researchers carried out extensive geographical mapping along with the diagnosis, age, knowledge, treatment, and medicinal plants' preparation methodologies. The identified 34 species, belonging to 23 families, were collected and placed in the national herbarium at the University of Abomey-Calavi in the Republic of Benin.[121] The researchers argued that of the 34 identified plants, *Ochna rhizomatosa* shrub (a.k.a bird's-eye bushes or Mickey-mouse plant) and *Ochna schweinfurthiana* (a.k.a Brick-red Ochna) were the ones the healers mentioned the most at 21%, followed by *Chasmanthera dependens* (a.k.a Chasmanthera or Ato-oloriraun) at 12%, *Piliostigma thonningii* (a.k.a monkey bread, camel's foot tree, or monkey biscuit tree) at 11%, and *Combretum sericeum* (a.k.a silky bushwillow) at 8%.[121] Coda Toafode et al. also pointed out that these five aforementioned plants were significantly noteworthy as they: "strengthened bones, reduced inflammation, relieved pain, and promoted healing" Coda Toafode et al.'s (2022), plus they held multiple (additional) purposes in the West African subregions.[121]

Although there are some new, high-tech methods of drug discovery currently (combinatorial chemistry, computer-based molecular modeling design), many drugs are made by "synthetic chemistry, none of them can replace the important role of natural products in drug discovery and development as most of the core structures or scaffolds for synthetic chemicals are based upon natural products," according to Veeresham.[118] And, in part, due to these new technologies, previously studied molecules are now adding new applications to their portfolios via enhanced modern molecular biology analyses and clinical observations.

Natural resources remain mankind's greatest source of novel structures as approximately half (85 of 175 molecules) of all approved drugs (1940s to date) were directly derived from nature.[122,123] Additionally, plant-derived compounds tend to have a more reliable reputation and history for effective patient tolerance. In 2001, Fabricant and Farnsworth reported that 80% of 122 plant-derived drugs were related to their original ethnopharmacological purposes, and current drug discovery relies heavily on bioactivity-guided fractionation (which have led to isolating many important anticancer drugs such as Paclitaxel [Taxol], Camptothecin, etc.).[123]

The first commercial natural product created for therapeutic use was morphine (sold by Merck in 1826); followed by the first semi-synthetic drug aspirin (from salicin isolated from *Salix alba*) sold by Bayer in 1899.[66] These discoveries led to the isolation of primary drugs like cocaine, codeine, digitoxin, quinine, and pilocarpine, some of which, in various forms, are still in use today. More recent plant-derived compounds that are on the pharmaceutical market include: Paclitaxel (from *Taxus Brevifolia*) for lung, ovarian, and breast cancer; Silymarin (from the seeds of *Silybum marianum*) for liver diseases; plant alkaloids that can be used in chemotherapy; Artemisinin, taken from the sweet wormwood plant (*Artemisia annua*) to combat multidrug-resistant Malaria; *Artemisia afra* (African Wormwood) was studied for COVID-19 and depression; and Trimesemine™, a monoamine-releasing agent is derived from the *Sceletium tortuosum*), or Kanna plant, is being studied for depression and Alzheimer's disease.[66] In the last decade, other plant-derived drugs include: Arteether (an antiparasitic medication derived from *Artemisinin*); Nitisinone (used to treat hereditary tyrosinemia type 1) derived from the Australian bottlebrush plant (*Callistemon citrinus*); Galantamine (an alkaloid extracted from the bulbs and flowers of *Galanthus nivalis, Galanthus caucasicus,* and *Galanthus woronowii*) is used to treat early stages of Alzheimer's Disease; and Cannabidiol from the cannabis plant (*Cannabis sativa*) and Capsaicin (from *Capsicum annuum*) used as pain relievers.[66]

High-tech conservation techniques, regulatory measures, and the ongoing revitalization of natural flora and fauna regions continually ushers in more and more novel challenges of quality control, research and development, standardization, and cost effectiveness in ethno-pharmaceuticals. So far, natural drugs have played an indispensable role in improving the human condition. Due to their safety and efficacy, they have proven, over and over again, to be the 'drug of choice' despite the onslaught of million-dollar, highly competitive mass-media marketing campaigns from computational/combinatorial chemistry compounds created at pharmaceutical giant laboratories. Perhaps the most remarkable characteristics of these natural-plant products is their richness in structural and functional diversity, species composition, and adaptation techniques—attributes, that to this day, remain largely unexplored, uncultivated, and untapped.

Medicinal Bonesetter Plants from Cameroon

As a nation, Cameroon has been dubbed 'Africa in Miniature' as it comprises approximately 90% of the African ecosystems: humid tropical forest, Sudan, the Sahelian (semi-arid steppe that lies just south of the Sahara), afro mountains, and mountain eco-regions—with a remarkable biological biodiversity of flora and fauna ranking fifth on the continent (after Congo, South Africa, Madagascar, and Tanzania).[3] This singular ethno-pharmacopoeia has been described as the "richest in Africa" according to researchers.[24,124] Some of the most commonly used flora and fauna include guava and pumpkin leaves, bitter kola, the *Dorstenia mannii* (Moraceae) plant, mashed guava leaves are traditionally used to alleviate pain, according to Makoge et al., as well as '*okongobong*' (fluted pumpkin leaves) and bitter kola (*Garcinia kola*), an indigenous flowering plant that produces large orange fruits and brown, nut-like seeds used in African ethno-medicine for coughs, colds, liver disease, etc.[58] The plant *Dorstenia mannii* (*Moraceae*) has been studied[125] and found to show significant antibacterial properties.

In a very specified study on bone regeneration in 2012, Ngueguim et al. evaluated six Cameroonian herbal plants for their restorative properties in bones and bone fractures. Because the six plants—*Elephantopus mollis*, *Spilanthes africana*, *Urena lobata*, *Momordica multiflora*, *Asystasia gangetica*, and *Brillantaisia ovariensis*—have been/and are currently used in Cameroonian traditional medicine for the treatment of bone diseases and fracture repair, the researchers assessed the plant's efficacies on bone and marrow injuries.[126] The researchers from the aforementioned study concluded that ethanol extracts from *Elephantopus mollis* (a.k.a 'false tobacco') leaves and (to a greater extent) the whole plant of *Spilanthes africana* (a.k.a. the 'toothache plant') "accelerated the bone healing process" after bone and bone marrow injury, "promoted compact assembly" in mineralized tissue of calluses, and "stimulated osteoblast recruitment at the injury site."[126p337]

The Baka, who inhabit the Dja reserve of Cameroon, were found to share many common plants in the Guinean-Congolian forests, and some of the plants most utilized in this area's traditional remedies include: *Aframomum daniellii* (a.k.a. African cardamom), *Alchornea cordifolia* (a.k.a. Christmas bush), *Astonia boonei* (a.k.a. God's tree—or in the Ghanaian Twi language '*Onyame dua*' or 'Tree of God'), *Carica papaya*, *Erythrophleum suaveolens* (a.k.a ordeal or sasswood tree), and *Pycnanthus angolensis* (a.k.a. African nutmeg).[127] Three published Cameroon-based 'success stories' in medicinal plant research, and subsequent national pharmaceutical manufacture, include: 1) HEPASORTM an oral solution for viral Hepatitis manufactured by Lobothera Laboratory since 2007, which is made from the stem bark of *Enantia chlorantha*, also known as African yellow wood; 2) POLA-GASTRAL A-T-200TM, manufactured by Kamsu-Kom Laboratory, which uses *Emilia coccinea* (*Asteraceae*) also known as the scarlet tassel flower, to treat stomach ulcers and gastritis, and 3) GAMA syrup, manufactured by AFRICAPHARM, used for hemorrhoids.[3]

Sagnia et al.'s (2014) research investigated any antioxidant capacities and anti-inflammatory activities of ethanol extracts of leaves of *Cassia alata* (a.k.a. Senna alata, candle bush, craw–craw plant, acapulo, ringworm bush, or ringworm plant), *Eleusine indica* (a.k.a Indian Goosegrass), *Carica papaya*, *Eremomastax speciosa*, and the stem bark of *Polyscias fulva* (a.k.a. the parasol tree) were all accumulated in Cameroon.[128] *Cassia alata* showed the highest antioxidant activity, according to the 2014 study. Antioxidants can be used to fight against cellular and tissue damage (caused by oxidative stress); these elevated levels of free radicals have been shown to contribute to AIDS, carcinogenesis (cancer), liver damage, inflammatory diseases, cataract formation, Alzheimer's disease, and many other diseases.[130,132-134]

Another 2015 study by Vij and Prashar concurred with Sagnia et al.[128] study, stating that *Carica papaya* possessed beneficial 'anti-inflammatory' as well as 'antimicrobial' properties, both useful in fracture care. The aforementioned study also reported that the papaya's enzyme 'papain' specifically can aid in the "treatment of traumas [...] and sports injuries."[128p3] Using an aqueous extract, which is a method of extracting active ingredients from plant matrices using water as a solvent) showed a significant 77% reduction in the wound area when compared to 59% contraction to wound of the controls; thus, the result suggested that the aqueous extract of *C. papaya* had a "potent wound healing property,"[p3] according to Vij and Prashar.[129] And while inflammation is a normal physiological response to tissue injury—if it remains uncontrolled, it can lead to additional (and unnecessary) complications. At the injury site, an increase in blood vessel wall permeability followed by migration of immune cells can cause edema formation during inflammation.

Four additional plants from Cameroon were tested by in 2007 by Biapa et al. for their phytochemical and antioxidant (mitigating cell destruction) properties: *Amphimas pterocaroides* (a.k.a. Lati, Yaya, or white oak), *Harungana madagascariensis* (a.k.a. dragon's blood tree, orange-milk tree or Haronga), *Myrianthus arboreus* (a.k.a. giant yellow mulberry or monkey fruit), and the Jansa tree, or *Cussonia barteri* [*Araliaceae*]—with *Harungana madagascariensis* and *Amphimas pterocaroides* reporting the highest antioxidant potentials using hydrolysed extracts of each plant.[130]

The *Cufod* is more commonly known as "*edem iduodut*" or "*ndadad edem*" by Ibibio people in Nigeria, and as "African blood tonic" in Cameroon.[131] The leaves of this 'weed' are usually utilized via decoction or infusion or maceration. Nigerian ethnobotanical (cold maceration methodology) leaf studies of the *Eremomastax speciosa* by Onoja et al. reported significant ($P < 0.05$) anti-inflammatory and antinociceptive activities in the extract, with optimal activities produced at the dose of 100 mg/kg.[131]

Much of what the bonesetters do is apply poultices to the injured areas, oftentimes with some measure(s) of immobilization, splinting, and bandaging. The aforementioned poultices were specific combinations of roots and herbs and leaves from various trees and bushes that were dried and ground up and combined into a paste that would be applied to the injured areas and then bound up with natural substances such as banana leaves. These recipes for the different poultices were passed down along familial lines via generations, alongside training of the preparation of the different components of their poultice(s), and then assisting the 'instructor bonesetter' with the applications.

Ethiopian Bonesetter Plants and Herbs

According to the Ethiopian Biodiversity Institute (EBI), over 80% of Ethiopians depend on traditional medicine from 887 medicinal plant species, and more than 95% of traditional medicinal preparations in Ethiopia are made from plant origin.[135] Other research reports show even higher rates of traditional plant medicine usage (at 90% and more) in Ethiopia and Burundi.[66] The EBI notes that the majority of the medicinal plants used in Ethiopia are first herbs (271 at 30.5%), followed by shrubs (168 at 19%), trees (110 at 12.4%), 'climbers' or vines (74 at 8.3%), reeds (2 at 0.2%), and finally 262 medicinal plants deemed "unidentified" at 29.6%.[135] Of the aforementioned medicinal plants utilized in Ethiopia, 357 (40.2%) are categorized as 'wild', 89 (10%) are deemed 'cultivated', and 52 (5.9%) are classified as 'weeds'.[135]

Abebe and Ayhue reported that traditional medicine offers a "significant contribution"[111p1] in first-aid needs of the Bensa district community in Ethiopia. The researchers go on to claim that the "persistence and recognition of this indigenous knowledge is due to the limited access to modern healthcare facilities"[111p1]; and that recordkeeping of the medicinal plants and their documented uses is a "critical issue" in order to safeguard the loss of indigenous knowledge concerning medicinal plants—which supports not only the human health care system, but also livestock care (via ethno-veterinary services). Unfortunately, the incongruous mismatch in private proprietorship vs. public health ideologies may prove incompatible for any genuinely symbiotic alliance between traditional healers and Western botanists.

Ghanaian Bonesetter Plants and Herbs

Some bonesetter's resistance to share their learned knowledge of plant-based medicines is sometimes due to a belief that their healing is a hard-won "gift from the ancestors" (perfected via years of apprenticeship); therefore, many remain reluctant to share information with a researcher, "even if the sharing might benefit themselves or their communities."[4p4]

Here we will take a more in-depth scientific review of three of TBS Agyemin Boateng Daniel's six utilized plants (Ghanaian TBS previously mentioned in Chapter 3):

1. Badie—the Badie tree (*Bridelia ferruginea*) was used by Daniel in the creation of his *dufa*. We found two studies by Awodele[136] and Bakoma[137] that discovered no mortality in studies performed on rats, however

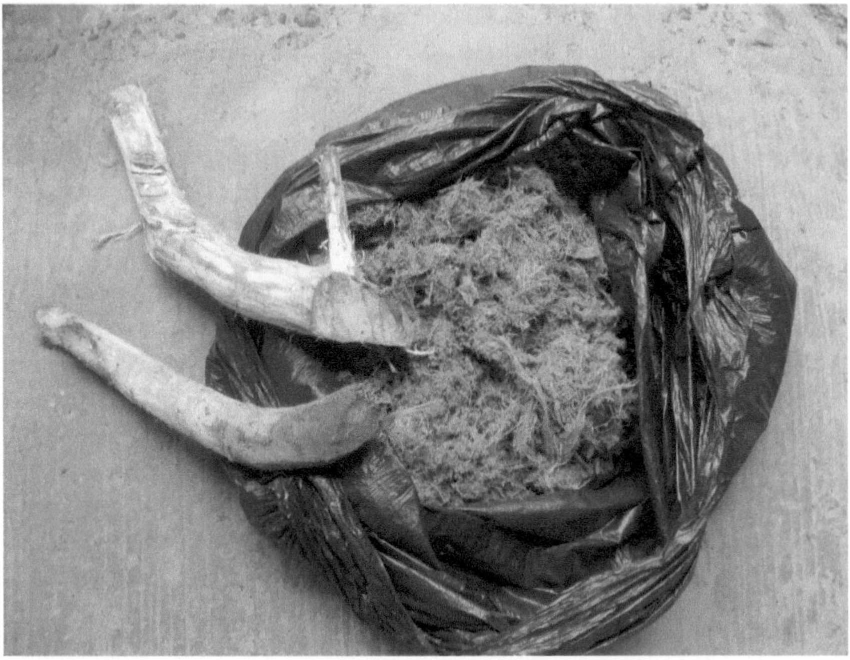

Photo 4.1. A traditonal bonesetter's amalgam of shaved plant mixtures that will be used as a poultice for external application on diseased and/or injured extremities.

Adwodele reported the ingested use of stem bark extract caused lipid peroxidation (which results in cell damage), as well as damage to sperm quality in studied male rats. Awodele noted that the stem bark extract "must be rarely used and if it's use is inevitable, antioxidant regimen must be incorporated."[136p9]

2. Kankan—fermented black garlic (*Allium sativum*) was also used by Daniel. Black garlic is merely regular garlic exposed to high humidity (70%–90%) and temperatures between 140° and 170° Fahrenheit for approximately 30–90 days. According to a food study by Kimura, properly fermented black garlic "exhibits several advantages when compared with fresh garlic."[138p68] Research has reported that fermented black garlic contains "more antioxidants than regular garlic,"[p68] as well as polyphenols, flavonoids, tetrahydro-β-carboline derivatives, and organosulfur compounds, including *S*-allyl-cysteine and *S*-allyl-mercaptocysteine.[139]

   In two other separate research studies by Aminuddin[140] and Kumar,[142] the researchers found that '*Kankan*' (in Twi Ghanaian language) showed various analgesic and beneficial motor-coordination properties. The two studies revealed that the plant was used for the treatment of mental and nervous system disorders in Ghana, and according to Amoateng, was an herb that had robust "scientific validation of their ethnopharmacological activities."[141]

3. Aboboma—also known as wild soursop or wild African custard-apple (*Annona senegalensis*).[252] In a recent Nugraha et al. study, extracts of Annona exhibited "moderate activities" against *Plasmodium falciparum*; methanol extracts of *Annona muricata* showed "apparent antimicrobial activities"; and alkaloids from Annona genus are "rich in structural diversity and pharmacological activities"[256] with the "potential for developing novel anti-infective and anticancer drugs."[143pl] In a 2011 study of *Annona senegalensis*, Ndjonka et al. reported the presence of flavonoids, alkaloids, saponins, carbohydrates, and tannins, and that these extracts "could provide alternatives in the control of helminthic infections."[144pl] The essential oil made from the wild soursop (steam distillation of dried leaves) was found to contain germacrene D (19.2%), β-caryophyllene (19.1%), γ-cadinene (11.1%), and α-humulene (9.7%) as its major components.[145]

What's in a '*Dufa*'?

The four aforementioned '*dufa*' samples were brought back to the United States—as the initial lab analysis performed by the Kwame Nkrumah University of Science & Technology scientists in Kumasi, Ghana, was disappointing. In Ghana, the scientists there could only ascertain that the samples were made up of unspecified 'biological materials'. Since the vast majority of the patients we interviewed were not only having these substances topically applied but were orally ingesting these herbal 'medicines' on numerous occasions (2–3 times weekly; based on the bonesetter's approved treatment regimen)—further studies into these unregulated and untested substances were warranted. However, the samples' American laboratory analysis included, but were not limited to, the following: to discern what organic elements are present in all four samples; to discern if any of the components present in the samples could be deemed harmful and/or detrimental to a person's health if orally ingested/consumed in certain quantities; and to test for and identify aerobic and non-aerobic bacteria, if any, that were present in the samples. Unfortunately, there was so much degradation of the unpreserved biological '*dufa*' samples, that no university laboratory analysis was successful in uncovering any specific substances we could definitively verify.

We also hypothesize that there will always be some percentage of 'unknown' findings as the TBS 'remedy' samples themselves were found left outdoors, in the open-air, and in dirty, unsterile environs. We witnessed firsthand that chickens and feral cats were seen walking, sleeping, and defecating on the bonesetter's drying 'medicine'—as well as being permeated with the naturally occurring insects, rodents, dust, dirt, and other contaminants that swirled nonstop around the outdoor samples. The names of these indigenous Ghanian plants are primarily in Twi (Ashanti region), but may be known by unfamiliar, indeterminate regional dialect/colloquial names—as the small West African nation (smaller than the state of Oregon, USA) boasts some 80 languages. It should also be noted that spellings of terms (cities, plants, places, etc.) throughout Ghana can take many different forms, and all are (seemingly) found to be acceptable and/or correct, especially in rural areas. Therefore, some of these spellings may be mispronounced or incorrectly spelled; all the bonesetters were without any formal education/illiterate or with only a primary education (semi-literate), so oral interpretations took precedence over any written communications. For a much more robust review of local Ghanaian names (in Twi, Dagomba, Fante, Konkomba, Dagomba, etc.), please review F.R. Irvine's (1961) book from Oxford University Press, "Woody Plants of Ghana"[146]; W.Hawthorne and N.Gyakari's (2006) book "Photo Guide for the Forest Trees of Ghana"[147] from the Oxford Forestry Institute (which details 326 trees, all with photos showing leaves, fruit, flowers, bark, wood and trunk and other identification aids; and R. Blench's "Dagomba Plant Names" (the language of north-eastern Ghana, Yendi, and Tamale areas).[148]

Four TBS 'Remedies'—Ingredients Uncovered

In addition to Daniel's samples, the second "*dufa*" sample, made by TBS Owusu-Sarpong, in the form of sun-hardened pellet, consisted of: ginger, water, roots of the Badie tree, bark and leaves of Kyerebentame; leaves from the 'elephant fighter' plant; roots from Brepun, and "*Efom wisa*" or black pepper. This bonesetter is not pictured in our text, but agreed to speak with us through an interpreter. Our third biological TBS sample was from Ghanaian teacher and apprentice, Adwoa Kuma and Peter Dwamena, from Akumsa Dumase. Their sample consisted of: *Akokomsuo* (unknown—Kuma warned to use roots only; and to never ingest); tree bark from Odum tree; leaves from basil '*Kokomo*'; and leaves from the Pawpaw (a.k.a. papaya). The pawpaw, or papaya (*Carica papaya*) leaf contains active components including alkaloids, glycosides, tannins, saponins, and flavonoids, and the juice of papaya leaves "increases the platelet counts in people suffering from dengue fever."[149p735] The same 2020 study concluded that the papaya leaf extract has "strong medicinal properties" including "antibacterial, antiviral, antitumor, hypoglycemic and anti-inflammatory activity."[149p735]

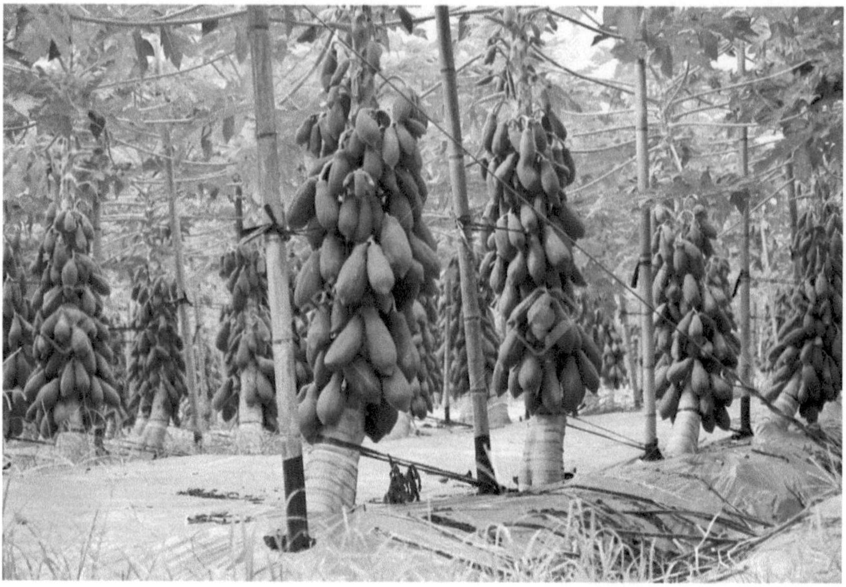

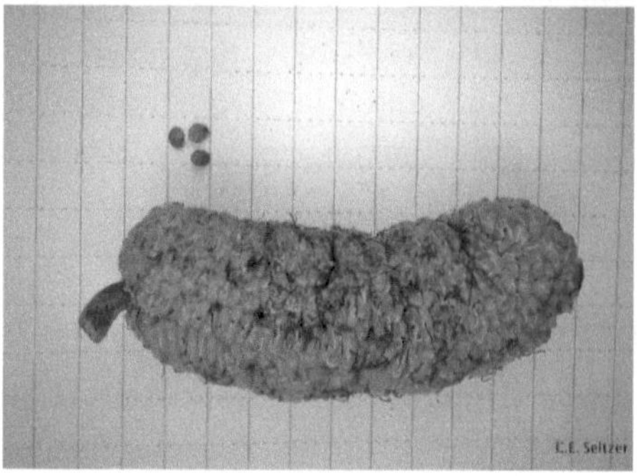

Photo 4.2–4.3. (Top) African Pawpaw. Photo credit: Oxfarm. (Bottom) *Odum* (*Milicia excelsa*) fruit and seeds. *Odum* is known as *'Abang'* in Cameroon *'Mvuli'* in Ethiopia, and is considered 'one of most powerful trees' in African herbalism. *Milicia regia* is one of two trees known as "*odum*" in Ghana, the other being the closely related *Milicia excelsa*. Photo credit: C.E. Seltzer.

In the nineteenth century, Bowdich (1966) collected 37 plants or "medicines [used] by the Ashantees."[150pl] Some of Bowdich's examples were for example: the cooked concoction of the bark of the '*Tandoorue*' (Tannuro—basil) tree and pepper was used for the relief of stomach pains and constipation; '*Bissey*' (Kola) was chewed (rather nonstop) by the Asante to "prevent hunger and strengthen the stomach and bowels"[150p371]; the crushed leaves of '*Anafranakoo*', were applied to boils, inflammatory swellings, and fractures as an advantageous all-natural remedy; the decoction (or the liquor resulting from concentrating the

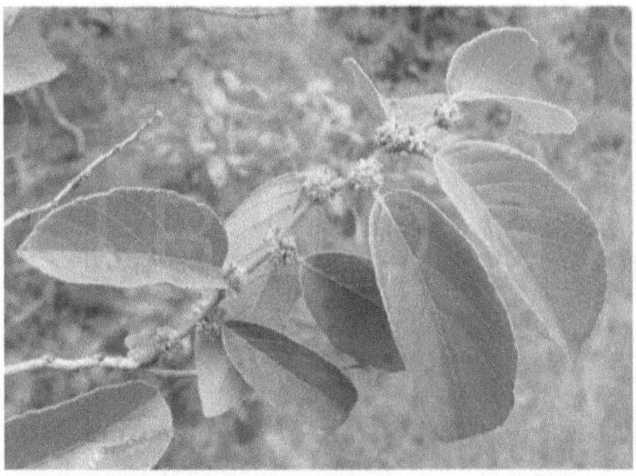
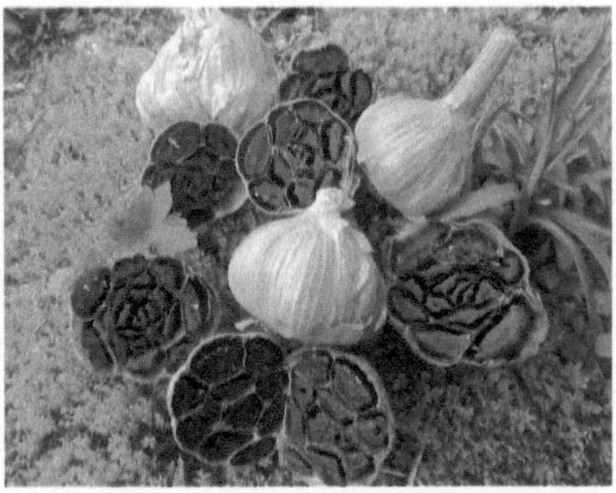

Photo 4.4–4.5. (L) Badie tree (*Bridelia ferruginea*) Photo credit: The Green Institute. (R) Fermented Black garlic or 'Gyene Kankan' (*Allium sativum*). Photo credit: The Green Institute.

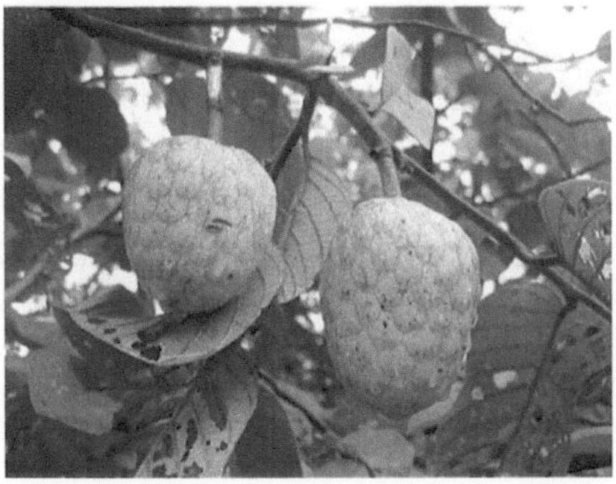
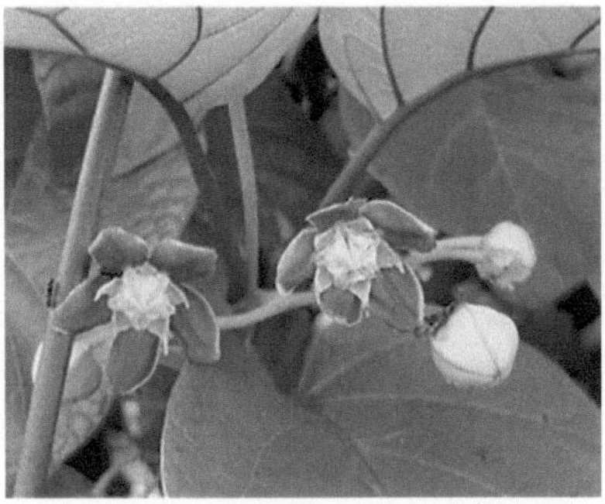

Photo 4.6–4.7. (L above) African Custard Apple (*Annona senegalensis*). Photo credit: Wikipedia 2020. (R above) Due to over-harvesting, *Mondia Whitei*, or white ginger root, is becoming endangered in several areas in Africa. Photo credit: Wikipedia 2024.

essence of boiling of the leaf) of the '*Kattacaiben*' (Kotodweben) was utilized for morning sickness among pregnant women; the bark of the '*Ocisseeree*' (Sisire/Kokonisuo) would ease vomiting among dysentery and diarrhea patients; and the '*Tointinney*' (Toantini, a.k.a. the "vein joiner" or *Paullinia pinnata*) herb, added to pepper, was considered a useful cough remedy[p377]. Bowdich offered that "even a child will easily list the medicinal uses of thirty or forty wild plants."[150p2]

Another important tree native to West Africa is the Bombax (*Bombax buonopozense*), a species that comes from the same family as the famous 'baobab' tree on the African savannas. Bombax trees have spikes growing on the bark, pink flowers, and seeds that produce 'kapok', a cotton wool-like material. The spikes on the bark are oftentimes burned into charcoal, which is used an anti-inflammatory. Yet another important tree from Ghana is the fast-growing

Emeri (*Terminalia ivorensis*). It is known to resist fungi and termites, so the bark extracts are used for yellow fever and rheumatism, as well as its anti-inflammatory and anti-arthritic properties. Yet another tree is the Mansonia (*Mansonia altissima*), or *Bété* or African Black Walnut. In Ghana and Nigeria, the tree is used for leprosy, syphilis, scabies, and yaws (a chronic skin infection with papillomas, or noncancerous lumps, and ulcers; caused by the bacterium *Treponema pallidum* subspecies *pertenue*, the same group that triggers venereal syphilis), according to a 2024 report from the WHO.[151] The last Ghanian tree of renowned local medicinal use is the Potrodom (*Erythrophleum ivorense*), that shows resistance to fungi, borers, and termites, so it is used locally for pain relief or as a laxative.

Zimbabwean Bonesetter Plants and Herbs

Ansellia africana (a.k.a. Leopard Orchid) is oftentimes used in traditional medicine as a love charm, an antidote for bad dreams, and at homes (to ward off lightning), according to the South Africa National Biodiversity Institute.[152] Portia, the Zimbabwean bonesetter (see Chapter 3) we interviewed for this book uses the green leaves of the *Anesellia* right when a patient first arrives to drink "so that the germs or infection will come out"—much like the prescribed regimen of antibiotics by Western-trained physicians. Intriguingly, this plant's ethnobotanical usage "has been documented in various traditional African pharmacopeias" and "has activity on the Central Nervous System" and "has shown potentiality in the treatment of

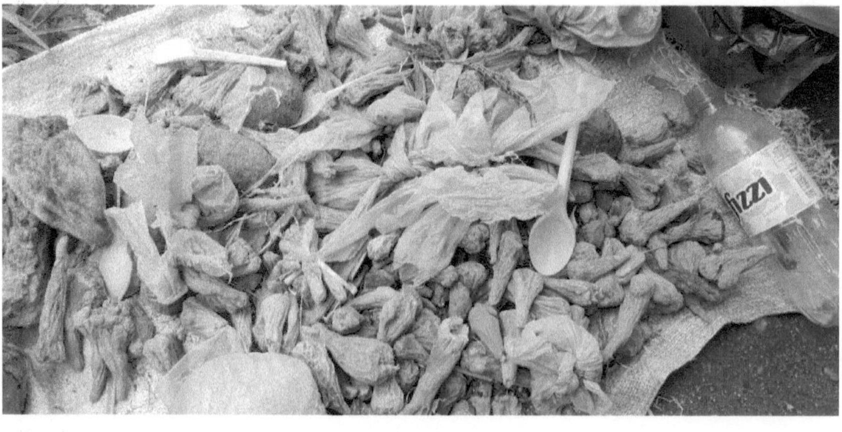

Photo 4.8. A Zimbabwean bonesetter's drying *Ansellia africana* Lindl. Family: Orchidaceae. Common names: leopard orchid (Eng.); *luiperdorgidee* (Afr.); *imfeyenkawu* (Zulu). Photo Credit: Wellington Mukwumbu, 2023.

Alzheimer's disease."[267p81] Another study claims that its stem infusions and smoke (from burning roots) are used by the Zulu as an antidote against bad dreams[154]; the leaves and stems make a drink potion for treating madness in Zambia[23]; and it is used as protective charm and aphrodisiac in Zimbabwe.[23] According to Chinsamy[155] research, it has "potent anti-acetylcholinesterase activity" and "can be used as an important source of various biomolecules for the treatment of Alzheimer's disease."[p88] However, due to over-exploitation and habitat destruction, this plant is facing the risk of extinction and has been categorized in the 'Red List of Threatened Species' as a 'vulnerable' plant by the International Union for Conservation of Nature and Natural Resources (IUCN).[156]

Perhaps one of the most recognized medicinal plants is the *Warburgia* (*Canellaceae*), a species that has a long history of ethnomedicinal uses in east, central, and southern Africa. Due to the popularity of *Warburgia* (a.k.a. "Pepperbark" or 'Wood Pepper") as a source of ethnomedicines, almost all of the species are severely over-harvested and 'vulnerable', according to the IUCN.[156] *Warburgia* species are used to treat everything from gastrointestinal disorders, colds, coughs, sore throat, fever, malaria, respiratory, and/or tooth/gum ailments, as they are abundant in *Drimane* and *Colorotane Sesquiterpenoides*, and other compounds.[156,157] The extracts of bark and leaves have shown pharmacological effects, including: antibacterial, antifungal, antimycobacterial, antioxidant, anti-inflammatory, antifeedant, antiplasmodial, antileishmanial, anthelmintic, cytotoxic (cell destruction), and molluscicidal (pesticidal) activities.[157,158] Traditionally, remedies produced from the *Warburgia* are well-known as a critical component among African traditional healing practices in the treatment of fungal, bacterial, and protozoal infections in both humans and animals, specifically 30 human and 7 animal ailments.[157,158]

Gather, Dry, Mash, Extract, and Store

At this time, it should also be noted that there are gathering, drying (or not), extraction, maceration, and/or storage techniques that alter phytochemical components utilized by TBS. According to Bird,[159] there are three main forms of extraction used for flowers, seeds, roots, leaves or berries: decoctions (an extraction made from roots, bark, or berries whereby ingredients are simmered over medium–low heat from 30 minutes to 5 hours); infusions (which are water-based teas or tisanes or brews, and oil-based infusions which sit in olive/sunflower/nut oil anywhere from four to six weeks); and tinctures, which are extractions from herbs using alcohol (such as vodka, grain alcohol, rum, or ethanol).

On an additional side note, a significant limitation of some of the aforementioned pharmacognosy, ethnobotanical, and phytochemistry studies noted in this book is the lack of a control group (a group that has no herbal remedy or takes a placebo, an inert substitute). This poses a patent dispute in any study using the scientific method, as any outcomes cannot be compared with those of the trial (herbal remedy) group. It should always be used to establish causality in phytochemistry studies of medicinal plants. A control population (group) allows scientists and physicians to determine that any change(s) observed in the 'active treatment group' was due to the herbal remedy being studied, rather than to other factors (like local-area pollution or malnutrition). Subsequently, there are five types of control groups, reports Oxford University's Critical Appraisal Skills Program, including (but not limited to) the following: 1) Concurrent placebo control (example = Group A gets the herbal remedy, but Group B gets an inert placebo); 2) Concurrent dose-comparison control (example = Group A gets a different dose than Group B of the same herbal remedy); 3) No treatment concurrent control (example = Group A gets herbal remedy, and Group B gets nothing—no placebo); 4) Concurrent active treatment control (example = Group A gets herbal remedy, but Group B gets a pre-existing herbal therapy that is known to be comparably effective); and 5) Historical control (patient data from previously treated or treated in a different setting(s) is utilized).[160] The robustness of any scientific study or experiment of native African medicinal plants lies in its reproducibility, followed by the subsequent logical analysis of the ascertained results.

That all being said, it can, in fact, still prove difficult to demonstrate the apples-to-apples comparability of patients in treatment and control groups. Given the rationale of a control group, it is critical that patients in both groups be of similar (baseline characteristics) like age, sex, and health. This is always easier said than done in clinical trials and medical investigations. As a researcher, imagine trying to locate a pool of 'clinical homogenous patients' with the exact same age, sex, disease(s), weight, medication and vitamin intake, geographical neighborhood, drinking, eating, and smoking habits, disease etiology, trauma severity, treatment history, presence/non-presence of comorbidities, concomitant exposures, and genetic variants [...]. Impossible! However, homogeneity (a measurement that supports the uniformity of subjects or variables), "is instrumental in minimizing variance, thereby enhancing the internal validity of studies that aim to research the efficacy of a specific intervention within a narrowly defined population," states Oxford University's Critical Appraisal Skills Program.[160] Thus, homogeneity in real-world clinical settings, strives to isolate specific patient characteristics (such as male patients between the ages of 25 and 30 with a bone density test result of a *T*-score of −1 or higher) that are consequential to that particular bone fracture healing study specifically. Perhaps Torday and Baluška[161] wrote on the importance of control groups in the methodologies, implementation, and publication of robust, controlled clinical trials best:

> Empirical research is based on observation and experimentation. Yet, experimental controls are essential for overcoming our sensory limits and generating reliable, unbiased and objective results…Beyond the methodology, controlling an experiment is critically important to ensure that the observed results *are not just random events*; they help scientists to distinguish between the 'signal' and the background 'noise' that are inherent in natural and living systems.[p10]

Here is a simplified example of how a clinical medicinal bonesetter plant trial can, quickly and inadvertently, become biased, and futile, pseudo-scientific dross: If an untreated (control) group consists of more aged women (with thin, weakened, Osteopenia, or Osteoporotic bones) than the other (treated herbal remedy) group of primarily 30-year-old men—the (incorrect and skewed) 'False-Positive' impression would be that the herbal remedy was extremely effective in bone healing; whereas the overlooked variable(s) of aged, thinned, and weakened bones of the elderly women vs. healthier bone structure and faster healing times of younger males—was unheeded. As you can well surmise, the failure to use a control group in any plant analysis (or the use of an inappropriate control group), can make it impossible to draw meaningful suppositions from any study—and lead to false conclusions, unreliable data, and/or inconclusive findings.

Some of these aforementioned plants must be rigorously studied to validate their phytoconstituents, bioactive compounds, and pharmacological activities and uses. The authors believe these studies are important because they validate the use of local pharmacopeia which might share related properties (which healers like Pa Tamnjong and others) might have used. We want to stress that we are extrapolating from these studies a universal rationale that the treatment of bone fractures constitutes a scientific practice, in that healers have studied local plants that have potent medicinal ingredients to effect healing of wounds and fractures. These results confirm the need for documenting traditional knowledge since it represents an opportunity for exploring plant species with pharmacological effects, which have, by and large, been (purposefully or not) excised from well-heeled corporate funding, monied pharmaceutical grants, and scientifically credible global investigations.

Adverse Side Effects

In conclusion, we would be remiss as scientists, researchers, and physicians to conclude this phytochemistry chapter without acknowledging the numerous possible adverse side effects of botanical preparations—including (but not constrained to): a potential for misidentification of poisonous plants; harmful interactions between some botanicals and conventional drugs, foods, or nutrients; overdose potential in under-regulated botanicals; and finally, "variation(s) in phytochemical constituents which depend on the stage of vegetative growth, part of the plant collected, soil type, plus other climatic factors."[41p61]

In a comprehensive meta-study of 492 scientific reports (Di Lorenzo et al.) published in the *British Journal of Clinical Pharmacology*, adverse effects were reported in 39 of the 66 studied botanical substances.[162] It is interesting to note some of 'top toxics' of the aforementioned study were soybeans at 19.3%, licorice at 12.2%, green tea at 8.7%, followed by gingko at 8.5% (86.6% of toxicities were associated with 14 plants).[162] Di Lorenzo's report also stated that 81.7% of adverse reactions could be directly associated with the botanical, 18.1% concerned interactions with medication, and one case was due to misidentification.[162] Certainly, direct causality assessments of any adverse botanical usages can prove a convoluted path. Unfortunately, the path of botanical over-/mis-use has led to concrete studies confirming a few noteworthy side effects: allergic reactions and hormone-like activities (from soybeans), hypokalemia and hypertension (from licorice), hepatotoxicity of *C. sinensis* (from green tea); abuse for adrenergic amines (from bitter orange, *C. aurantium*); head, neck, mouth, esophageal cancer (from chewing native Betel nuts),[253] and many more.[162,255,257–259]

Of course, it is quite possible that we, as a global scientific community, continue to underestimate adverse side effects of all-natural botanicals, as people generally consider flora and fauna as harmless, all-natural and fundamentally 'safe' components (and don't report their use to healthcare practitioners); therefore, data collection on harmful or fatal botanical usage(s) by poison centers reports is a relatively small, and usually only published concerning acutely excessive (or fatal) vitamin/mineral/botanical cases. Our next chapter will take us back in history, in fact, all the way back to the very beginnings of bone-setting treatments.

Chapter 5

A BRIEF GLOBAL OVERVIEW INTO THE DEVELOPMENT OF ORTHOPEDIC SCIENCE

The word orthopedics, which was coined in 1741 by Nicholas Andry, was derived from Greek words "*orthos*" for "correct" or "straight" and "*paidon*" for "child."[163p59] This was developed from the knowledge of the process of traditional bone-setting where a splint made of bamboo is tied round the particular limb in order to immobilize the fractured limb. Throughout history, limb fractures have been treated via an enormous array of handcrafted, cobbled-together, or specialty manufactured immobilization, traction, amputation, and/or internal fixation materials. Immobilization—either via casting, bracing, or splinting—a joint above and below the fracture is used for most long-bone fractures, except in the case of femoral fractures (traction is mainstay of treatment). Unfortunately, in the past, open fractures and ballistic wounds associated with long-bone fractures were not too responsive to available medications (due to associated soft-tissue injury and the difficulty of preventing sepsis), so amputation was seen as the safest and most convenient alternative at the time.

As we will see, the development of medicine and surgery in Europe, Asia, Great Britain (and later in the Americas) differed from African practices in some very important ways. Historically, the practice of ancient medical practitioners and modern African bonesetters hold distinct similarities—whereby practical, hands-on training in the use of herbal medicines and remedies are passed orally from father to son, or practitioner to apprentice; written theoretical textbooks are not in evidence. There is no 'collaborative' atmosphere among African bonesetters that promotes teamwork or the sharing of knowledge, as each healer holds their secretive 'tricks of the trade', with lifelong financial incentives to (solely) develop their reputation while retaining their exclusive 'magical' secrecies. We can only begin to imagine the amount of 'uncaptured knowledge' in global ethnobotanical studies that has already been tragically lost forever.

In opposition to this rather tightlipped trickle-down training, was the European, Asian, and American establishment's public-domain usage of the Scientific Method, written textbooks, civic learning center formation, and the printing press. Noticeably, when societies choose to leverage their collective intelligence, they can omit duplicating time-consuming efforts, increase efficiencies and innovations, share painful 'lessons learned' know-how, and build communal trust in their professional and academic peers. When people do not feel safe sharing their ideas—or even perhaps more importantly—their mistakes, they are disinclined to form partnerships and unmotivated to use their valuable time and resources toward goals they do not understand, respect, or support.

When looking at the history of orthopedic care, we have to realize that it goes back to the beginning of history itself. Humans have been injuring themselves since we first appeared on earth. There were records of treatments for orthopedic injuries in the writings of the Egyptians. Historical scholars note that as early as 1600 B.C., a record was found with instructions on treating an upper-arm fracture, and in 1900 B.C., King Hammurabi recorded regulations concerning patient care practices, specifically noting that the '*Ghallabu*', or slave bonesetters, would conduct branding (of slaves), dental care, and minor surgeries.[164] In truth, the treatment of fractures and dislocations prior to the mid-1800s was nonoperative and consisted of manual reductions and immobilization using some sort of splint or immobilization substance.[165] Prior to the invention of anesthesia the only real orthopedic surgery consisted of amputations of limbs that had gotten infected or lost their circulation.

Before Hippocrates, the practice of medicine was saturated with local mysticism and illusory superstition. Orthopedics was no different. Hippocrates founded the school which bore his name, and his compendium Hippocratic Corpus, or '*Corpus Hippocraticum*', consisted of 60 books on various medical topics (diseases, childbirth, pediatrics, patient case histories, treatment regimens, wound, and fracture care, etc.), and was the first documented attempt to make a serious academic study of surgery, internal medicine, orthopedics, traumatology, and obstetrics—and to decisively delineate medical sciences from superstition, religion, and magic.[166] Two of the books had particular relevance to orthopedics, including "The Articulations" and "On Fractures."[166] Surgeons at that time were quite familiar with problems such as contractures, disuse atrophy, and pressure ulcers. In their writing there was no such thing as 'laudable pus' (suppuration that, at the time, was viewed as a sign of positive healing). Cleanliness was important, dressings were changed frequently and injured parts were put at rest. They developed a technique to prevent recurrent shoulder dislocations by scarifying the lax part of the shoulder capsule using a cautery introduced through the axilla.[167]

Hippocrates felt that disease was a disruption in the balance of the 'four humors of the body', consisting of: blood, phlegm, black bile, and yellow bile.[166] Other theories (what we now know as infectious diseases) included the idea of Miasma (the Greek word for "bad air") which was first proposed by Hippocrates.[166] The theory was that these 'bad humors' came from decomposing organic materials (plants or animals), which then, in turn, poisoned the air. This so-called 'bad air' was easily detectable due to noxious, rotting odors; therefore, people who kept inhaling 'bad air' would, logically, become ill from the stench. Some efforts to remove waste and maintain cleanliness were begun in order to maintain wellness and good health.

Galen (a.k.a. Aelius Galenus, Claudius Galenus, or Galen of Pergamon 129–200 A.D.) was a student of Hippocrates, served as a physician to the gladiators, and as such he would see the mutilated and slain bodies up close and was able to view (previously unobserved) anatomical bones, organs, and features.[167] Up until this time in history, no dissections of the human body were allowed which meant the internal anatomy of humans was largely a mystery. Galen is most famous for discovering the human 'pulse', blood movement via human arteries, and he is considered to be 'the greatest anatomist of antiquity and the founder of experimental physiology'—so while other physicians of his time were contemplating 'life spirit', he was describing neuromuscular control of voluntary muscle and the brain as the central regulating force of the neuromuscular system.[167] His writings (and its subsequent physiological and medical errors) dominated Western medical thought for some 1,000 years. Galen also extended the 'four humors' theory of Hippocrates so that each '*humour*' was ascribed to a season. At the time, people noticed that changes in the weather (via rain, heat, cold, etc.) would disrupt the balance of human '*humours*' (via fevers, Malaria, Salmonella, etc.) so blood-letting, enemas, and induced vomiting (purges) were considered good medical practices that persisted until the Germ Theory of Disease was accepted doctrine.

Even back in 400 B.C., Hippocrates' book 'On Fractures' keenly addressed 'excessive' tightness in compression bandaging, good blood flow (circulation), swelling (Compartment Syndrome), and proper healing of a hand/arm fracture (as translated by Francis Adams) below:

> And these are the signs that the patient has been well treated and properly bandaged: if you ask him if the arm feels tight, and he says it does, but moderately so, and especially about the fracture; and this reply he should make all along, if the bandage be properly applied. And these

> are symptoms of the bandaging being moderately tight; if for the first day and night he fancies that the tightness does not diminish, but rather increases; and if on the next day there be a soft swelling in the hand, for this is a sign of moderate compression, but at the end of the second day the compression should feel less, and on the third day the bandaging should appear loose. And if any of these symptoms be wanting, you may conclude that the bandaging is slacker than it should be; or if any of these symptoms be in excess, you may infer that the compression is more than moderate; and judging from these, you will apply the next bandages either slacker or tighter [...] When the third day arrives, that is to say, the seventh from the first dressing, if properly done, the swelling in the hand should be not very great; and the part which has been bandaged should be found more slender and less swelled at each time, and on the seventh day the swelling should be quite gone, and the broken bones should be more readily moved, and admit of being easily adjusted[166] (Excerpts from Parts 5 and 6).

About that same time, Hippocrates also invented a traction table called the '*Scamnon Hippocrates*' (a.k.a. the Hippocratic bench).[166] This flat wooden table was used to stretch out painful joints, discs, and tendons for back pain, the realign overlapping fractures, and curvature of the spine, etc. Interestingly, some less-than-constructive uses of the traction bench was to rework them into torture devices like the notorious 'rack'. Even today, modern orthopedic traction tables use analogous mechanisms constructed imitating this ancient design.

These copious writings by Hippocrates served as the dominant source of medical knowledge for 500 years[167]; during this time theoretical knowledge and logic ruled supreme, so practical aspects of hands-on corporal experimentation were deemed unnecessary. Indeed, up until now, there were no firsthand visual/physical explorations (via dissection) into anatomical structures, spatial relationships, and functioning of organs and tissues.

In 350 B.C., Hippocrates wrote of wrapping injured limbs in cloth bandages soaked in wax and resin. According to the 'Edwin Smith Surgical Papyrus' (Circa 1500 B.C.), Egyptians were using self-setting bandages for fracture management.[168] What was particularly fascinating about this ancient text was that there was a 'diagnosis section' where he categorized each case within three verdicts: (1) "[This is] a medical condition I can heal"; (2) "[This is] a medical condition I intend to fight with"; and (3) "[This is] a medical condition that cannot be healed."[168p1817] Much like modern-day triage assessments, this therapeutic reasoning showed that this Egyptian physician had treated many traumatic injuries.

Old World Medicine

The large medical institutions (that we are familiar with today) were just beginning to be established, subsequently in the 1100s–1200s many of the original European medical schools were created (like the University of Paris in 1110, Bologna in 1113, Oxford in 1167, Montpellier in 1181, Padua in 1222, and Naples in 1224), signal all of which signaled the end of the medieval epoch and the start of the Renaissance.[169] King Roger of Sicily was the first to require certification for the practice of medicine in 1140. At Bologna, the study of anatomy was enhanced when Emperor Frederick II allowed, and then compelled, dissection of humans in Italian medical schools. These post-Renaissance schools relied on empirical observation or "seeing to believe."[169pl]

Much like the current chasm between traditional bonesetters and physicians today, there had been a historical dichotomy between a 'Physician' and a 'Surgeon' in medicine. Historically, physicians were viewed as the hyper-educated, university-trained specialists, whereas surgeons were merely barbers that accompanied armies to treat wounds. In the time of Homer, surgeons were called "*Iatros*" which meant "remover of arrows."[169pl] It seems as though the 'manual nature' of surgical work was considered more of a trade (thus unacceptable for university study)—whereby the belief was "there [was] no more science in surgery than in butchering."[169pl] Still today, the cooperation between surgical and medical specialists is sometimes tentative and rather punitive based on the two uncompromising systems of approaches to disease/injury treatment(s).

It was not until the sixteenth century via the work of John Hunter and Ambrose Pare that the status of the 'surgeon' became to be recognized as a profession on par with the physician.[169] They also were able to replace a thousand years of cumbersome splints and braces which much simpler, lightweight devices. This culminated with the work of Pare on brace-making techniques. Guy de Chuliac, Professor of Surgery at Montpellier, France, devised the traction-suspension method for the treatment of femoral (the body's longest bone) fractures.[169]

Down through history medical advances seemed to parallel advances in war as the need for treating the different types of war wounds exponentially increased. In 1331, firearms were developed, closely followed by the battlefield cannon around 1346. These new weapons created a whole new class of war injuries—with more devastating destructions to human flesh and bone. In 1450, the establishment of the printing press suddenly made medical textbooks available to large numbers of physicians and the dissemination of advances; whereas previously, lengthy academic texts needed to be hand-copied.[169]

In the fifteenth and sixteenth centuries, human anatomy—as an art and science—trans-morphed into a dynamic, functional discipline with advances made by the notable likes of Leonardo Da Vinci and Vesalius. In 1543, Vesalius published his "*De Fabrica Humani Corporus*", establishing him as the greatest anatomist of his time.[169] A barber-surgeon (which was a standard job for the time) to several European monarchs, named Ambrose Pare, made many contributions to the medical and surgical communities at large. Perhaps most notably, Pare popularized the use of ligatures made of silk thread to stop bleeding, rather than practicing the age-old cauterization. Finally, the discovery of the 'circulation of the blood' by William Harvey in 1628, supplanted the erroneous Galenic concepts of circulation—which would have a deep-rooted effect on wound healing.[170] This momentous medical discovery will be discussed next.

Circulation of the Blood

The discovery of the circulation of the blood was attributed to William Harvey, an English-born physician who became a Fellow of the College of Physicians at St. Bartholomew's Hospital, lecturer at the College of Physicians, and later, in 1618, he was appointed as personal physician to King James The First.[170] Harvey's medical contemporaries, according to Ribatti,[170] believed that heart's primary function was the production of heat, and blood was thought to be constantly consumed in the periphery and replenished by ingested nutrients (which was carried out by the right ventricle and 'great veins'). At the time, there was not any physiological connection from the arteries and veins (capillaries). However, Harvey discovered that the valves of the heart only allow the blood to flow in one direction—and he demonstrated that the heart pumps blood to the lungs with the right side, back to the heart, and out to the body—postulating that the presence of capillaries or ('pores in the flesh') allowed the blood to return to the heart via the veins.[170] It was that eureka moment that led Harvey to conclude that blood moves around the body in a circle that moves continuously. It was not until the invention of the microscope that the existence of capillaries could be proven; the existence of which were purely theoretical during Harvey's lifetime.

Fast Doesn't Always Mean Good

At University College Hospital in central London in the early 1840s, surgeon Robert Liston was famous for his ability to remove a patient's leg in 25 seconds, as reported the BBC in 2020.[171] Notorious for his speed, high intensity, and success rate—a Liston amputation had a 1:6 fatality rate—far lower than other

Victorian surgeons, the BBC report by R. Hollingham in 2020 noted.[171] As there was no pain relief, his swift cutting lessened the exposure time of tissue to microbes and infection, as well as shortening the (almost unimaginably) horrific trauma of surgery for the patient who was held down on a wooden bench by assistants. Unexpectedly, during one amputation, Liston cut through his assistant's fingers, and, with that, an observer in the room died on the spot from shock, plus the patient and the surgical assistant later died of infections—making it "probably the only operation in history with 300% mortality,"[pl] as Hollingham noted.[171] If nothing else, medical history is filled with tales of the wry, the tragic, and the patently absurd.

War-Time Sawbones: "He Who Wishes to Be a Surgeon Should Go to War"

During the American Civil War, doctors were easily recruited to their relevant native armies, as the training was far more hands-on and comprehensive than what was offered during an apprenticeship of the 'physician-to-be' with a more experienced physician. Even Hippocrates said: "He who wishes to be a surgeon should go to war."[166] From all accounts, long-term career army surgeons had little concern, time, or sympathy for the medical volunteers who were unprepared for the horrific bloodshed and battlefield conditions during the American Civil War. As one example, the war's novel use of the soft-lead 'Minié Ball' (named after Claude-Etienne Minié) was enormous when considering a soldier's physiological gunshot wound trauma.[165] The infamous 'Minié Ball',upon impact flattened the top of its cone out, resulting in acute tissue destruction and splintering of bone. The vast majority of wounds documented during the Civil War were caused by the Minié ball, tragically instigating about 75% of battle-related surgeries to result in amputations.[165] Frequently, battlefield surgeons moved swiftly from war casualty to war casualty, performing amputations using the same saw, hence the moniker 'Sawbones' being given to the tool-wielding practitioners.[165]

'Good and Laudable Pus' vs. Germ Theory

The 'Germ Theory of Disease' wasn't widely recognized until after the American Civil War (1861–1865). In fact, it used to be assumed that having pus draining from a wound was a beneficial sign of healing—so it was dubbed as 'Laudable Pus'.[172] Consider for a moment if you will, that after arduous examinations, skillful imaging, and research, you have reached a solid diagnosis for your patient. Then you successfully complete a long, meticulous, even miraculous, reconstructive surgery [...] but during the recovery period, the patient's operative site becomes infected, the patient becomes septic [...] and dies. This scenario serves to illustrate the consequence(s) of the Germ Theory of Disease—and why modern methods of antisepsis, sterile technique, cleansing of wounds, and the use of antibiotics play such a vital role in patient care.

So, it really wasn't that long ago (in the eighteenth and nineteenth centuries) that the 'Germ Theory of Disease' was pioneered. Before that, the idea that tiny organisms—invisible to the human eye—could possibly invade the body and cause disease was neither believable nor plausible. Lauded as the 'most important discovery in the history of medicine' by many, the Germ Theory ushered in a quantum shift in the way people thought about disease, and for the first time, separated the disease from the patient.

Another misconception (often blamed on Galen) was the idea of so-called 'laudable pus'.[265] This old-world belief was that the presence of pus was beneficial for wound healing and should be encouraged. This misconception probably relates to the fact that chronic wound infections produce thick whitish yellow pus; while necrotizing infections (despite their severity and high mortality) are usually devoid of pus. In part, due to this misconception, the idea of "good and laudable pus"[165] was, to the misfortune of man, accepted dogma among surgeons for centuries to follow.

Puerperal Fever

Consider what many regard as the 'sad story' of medical pioneer Dr. Ingaz Semmelweis. He was working as an obstetrician at the University of Vienna hospital when he witnessed an outbreak of Puerperal Fever (childbed fever)—which had a very high mortality rate at the time.[172] The university's maternity clinic had two divisions: Division One was where medical students were taught; Division Two was where midwives worked. He noted that mortality rates from Puerperal Fever was three times higher in Division One.[172] Sadly, at that time, 'Childbed Fever' was running rampant across all European maternity clinics. Dr. Semmelweiss contemplated many causes, but it wasn't until his close friend, forensic pathologist, Professor Jakob Kolletschka accidentally cut his finger during an autopsy, developed sepsis, and died that the connection was made.[172] Dr. Semmelweis examined autopsy findings and concluded that they were identical with the mothers who were dying from Puerperal Fever.[172] He inferred that 'cadaveric particles' were introduced into his blood stream via a cut, however, he was also aware that physicians-in-training moved straight from autopsies to the delivery room—without washing their hands. At that, he began requiring all students to wash their hands using an extremely stringent solution—and consequently, the incidences of puerperal fever dropped dramatically.[172]

Regrettably, the medical students and doctors balked at washing their hands with this harsh solution. The doctors felt like Semmelweiss put them at fault, so they kicked him out of the hospital. The medical doctors returned to their prior practices and Puerperal Fever skyrocketed again. Defeated, Semmelweiss returned to his homeland of Hungary, suffered a mental breakdown, and tragically ended up in an insane asylum. Two weeks later, he was wounded in a fight, developed a wound infection, and (quite ironically) died of sepsis.[172]

The reality that doctors could be functioning as 'unwitting vectors of disease' was not only shocking and professionally controversial, it also began a distressful ripple effect throughout the medical field. However, this theory remains germane even today, as many traditional African bonesetters who unwisely treat open fractures in dirty, unsterile outdoor environs (via unwashed hands and rusty implements), put their patients at high risk for developing deadly infections.

It wasn't until the invention of the microscope in the seventeenth century that the existence of these teeny-tiny microorganisms could be confirmed, commencing the historic study of Bacteriology. Antonie Von Leeuwenhoek was credited with this invention and was later dubbed the 'Father of Microbiology'. Nonetheless, even though the scientific community could now view these tiny creatures, it did not mean that the ever-resistant 'House of Medicine' was going to speedily jump on board. The idea was met with significant resistance: One had to prove causation [...] And what if these miniscule microorganisms were not pathogenic?

Pasteur and Lister

This all happened a few decades before Louis Pasteur and Lister came to fame. They were visionaries, however, and recognized the importance of Semmelweis' work. The two built upon his work to create a more complete set of antiseptic techniques. Pasteur was able to show that germs were causing infection delivering the missing pieces of information needed to make antisepsis widely accepted. Pasteur was a scientist who discovered that microorganisms caused fermentation—and that boiling stopped the process, killing the bacteria.[173] This led to the creation of the process called 'Pasteurization'.[173]

Lister showed that using carbolic acid to sterilize instruments and to put in wounds intraoperatively before closure (suturing) significantly reduced postoperative wound infections.[173] It was during the mid-1800s that Lister introduced open reduction and internal fixation (ORIF) of patella fractures in the 1860s, the use of plates, screws, and wires was first documented in the 1880s and 1890s.[165] In 1865, the consensus was that an open fracture needed to be treated with amputation to prevent death from infection. Dr. Lister, who didn't believe in 'laudable pus' was presented with an 11-year-old boy with and open fracture of his left lower leg.[173] He used primitive disinfection with cloth soaked in acid, set and splinted the wound—and six weeks later the boy was completely healed.[173] This led to the conclusion that pus was not only bad, but that it was preventable. While this theory became the general consensus in the United Kingdom and Europe, the American medical establishment was more recalcitrant and skeptical to adopt the theory. So, in 1876, Lister came to the United States and lectured to more than 500 physicians in Philadelphia about his success with infection-free wounds.[173] His reception was met with skepticism (even though by then he had robust statistics to support his theory). Physicians, historically, have possessed a rather notorious resistance to change. So, it wasn't until 1879 that the first 'antiseptic surgery' in America was performed in Boston. In the 1890s (partially due to the death of an American President), 'Listerism' (the antiseptic surgical method that utilizes a carbolic acid solution) was applied to surgery in America.[173]

Thus began the modern age of antisepsis. Everything that has happened since still stands stalwartly on these cornerstone principles. The theory of antisepsis is applicable to all types of surgery, including orthopedics.

Fracture Reduction

The art of reduction was basically an attempt to make the injured extremity look like the patient's (other) uninjured extremity. Before the invention of modern pain medicines and sedatives, this would have been an agonizingly painful endeavor. The importance of circulation to an injured extremity has been an enduring discovery. In the first half of the eighteenth century, the custom was to wait until swelling had substantially decreased enough to reduce a broken bone. Joseph Sampson Gamgee (1828–1886), a surgeon at the Queen's Hospital, developed surgical dressings and an early modern technique of fracture reduction.[169]

Those Glowing 'X'-Rays

After fracture reduction, the other scientific development that really brought Orthopedics into the modern era was the advent of X-rays. Miraculously, the anatomy of bones could be visualized—including damage(s) inflicted via trauma—without first surgically cutting the patient open. Plus, more specific injuries could be identified and attempts to correct them could be evaluated visually. Prior to the advent of X-rays, the best outcome of a closed reductions was via 'visual observation', or to, simply put, make the injured side look like the other (uninjured) side.

The development of X-rays to diagnose orthopedic injuries did not even exist prior to the twentieth century. Some time on November 8, 1895, Wilhelm Conrad Röntgen discovered that shining a cathode ray through a glass of water led to a glow coming from a chemically treated screen. He called them 'X-rays' due their unknown nature, according to the European Society of Radiology.[174] Röntgen discovered that these mysterious 'rays' could penetrate many types of matter, including human flesh. He soon took an X-ray of his wife's hand which showed the bones and the wedding ring. Two years later, the first documented use of X-rays on a military battlefield was utilized to search for bullets and broken bones. Six years after Röntgen noticed the glow of X-rays, he received the first-ever Nobel Prize in physics.[174] Even though the discovery of X-rays was a major milestone in the history of modern medicine, Röntgen never sought any exclusive rights to sell or to patent the public's free application of X-rays into the fields of medical imaging, materials analysis, and the study of the structure of matter.

With the invention of radiology, medical doctors now had the ability to use a noninvasive technique to see inside the human body. This was a paradigm shift in medicine. However, there were also casualties along the way—with early pioneers dying of radiation poisoning—like Clarence Dally, Thomas Edison's assistant (who died of metastatic melanoma) after working extensively with X-rays.[174] X-rays went on to became somewhat of a 'newfangled' irradiating American curiosity of the time. From 1930s through the early 1950s, shoe-fitting X-rays fluoroscopes (a.k.a. the X-rays Shoe Fitter, Pedoscope, and Foot-o-scope) were used in 10,000 U.S. stores, 3,000 U.K. stores, and 1,000 Canadian stores, but this unnecessary radiation exposure was stopped after Dally and many others died from overexposure to radiation.[174] Also, the initial limitations of the technology caused difficulties, as patients had to remain still for several minutes in order to get a useful image. So, if you were attempting a chest X-ray, a single breath would have ruined the entire image. Nonetheless, over the years, many improvements led to shorter X-ray times and cut down on doses/exposure to radiation. Today, one of the ways to enhance X-ray imaging is through use of oral contrast media, which is radio-opaque (showing internal organs), or via IV injection (showing circulation between and within internal organs).

However, with the advent of the computer age, suddenly the idea of using computers to form much more complex images led to the development of computerized tomography or CT's, ultrasounds, and MRIs which is where we are today. When compared to modern medicine (with all of our state-of-the-art imaging technologies), it is incomprehensible to imagine how orthopedic surgeons in the distant past (with no imaging technologies) were able to assess and successfully operate on their injured patients [...] without the indomitable X-ray. Of course this was just the beginning. The very early techniques of radiography have been modified and refined. The risk of radiation exposure has led to techniques to lower exposure to radiation while improving the scanned images, leading to the creation of noninvasive, state-of-the-art modalities such as positron emission tomography (PET), ultrasonography, computerized axial tomography (CAT), single-photon emission computed tomography (SPECT), and magnetic resonance imaging (MRI) which is used today, and artificial intelligence (AI) in medical imaging which will be in used in the future.[174] The detailed, high-quality, cross-sectional, and/or 3-D aspects possible with these low-risk, noninvasive imaging technologies has completely transformed what is possible for orthopedic surgeons to realize today.[174]

Computed tomography scans, that utilize X-rays for cross-sectional images, were not developed until the 1980s and magnetic resonance imaging (MRI) (uses magnetic fields and radio waves to build image of internal structures).[174] Before these (imaging technologies that we rely on so heavily today) all diagnoses were accomplished by clinical observation and visual examination.

Antibiotics

If a fracture is open (a wound in the skin that 'communicates' with the fracture), the risk of infection is much greater. Proper modern treatment of an open fracture involves taking the patient to the operating room, and performing a debridement (or washing out) the wound to try to get all the germs, bone fragments (if any), and debris out in order to stave off possible infection. Antibiotics may be used prophylactically in this situation. Many times, the wounds are not closed for a few days to prevent the development of osteomyelitis (infection of the bone). Again, before the advent of modern anesthesia, the capacity to perform this surgery would have been nearly impossible. It's also important to consider that a bone fracture may also accompany other surrounding injuries (internal muscle damage, fractured spleen, etc.) and the patient's comorbidities should be considered (and how they might interfere with proper healing).

Advent of Anesthesia

Now we have discussed the various imaging technologies that have emerged, as well as antibiotics. However, prior to the advent of anesthesia, sophisticated and complex surgeries were considered impossible, as the patient would be moving, screaming, and writhing in pain. Therefore, the majority of orthopedic surgeries for injuries (before anesthesia) were fast amputations. By and large, one of the most important developments in the history of medicine (in general) and orthopedics (in particular) was the development and evolution of anesthesia. Orthopedic injuries by their very nature tend to be painful and any attempt to manipulate or do surgery on such an injury will also be very painful. This limited what could be done to surgically uncomplicated procedures like amputations.

According to the Wood Library Museum of Anesthesiology in Schaumberg, Illinois, USA, documented attempts to alleviate patient's pain go back as far as 4,000 years B.C., with evidence of the use of the opium poppy in Sumerian texts, followed by the Babylonians use of Henbane (*Hyoscyamus niger*, a.k.a. black henbane or stinking nightshade, is a toxic plant containing atropine, scopolamine, and hyoscine) to relieve toothaches around 2,250 B.C.; Inca shamans were known to chew coca leaves and drip their cocaine-laden saliva into the wounds of patients; and acupuncture in 1,600 B.C. in the Shang Dynasty in China.[175] Though the application of carotid pressure was also utilized to induce unconsciousness for circumcision and eye surgery around 400 B.C.E. by the Egyptians and Assyrians.[175] For several hundred years, people used various concoctions of herbal remedies, as well as opium, to induce a 'soporific state' by instilling the different concoctions onto a sponge and dripping them into the patient's nostrils.[175]

The first use of modern ether anesthesia was implemented on animals by Paracelsus in 1525, and in 1659, the pioneering use of intravenous injection was accomplished using a goose quill to inject opium into a dog's vein, according to the Wood Library.[175] Then, in 1805, pharmacist Frederick Sertürner took an extract of opium, named Morphium (after Greek god of dreams, Morpheus) for use as an anesthetic; later, in 1846, the first surgery using ether anesthesia was conducted at Massachusetts General Hospital whereby a neck tumor was removed painlessly by Dr. John Collins Warren.[175]

The list of anesthesiologic inventions goes on and on [...]. Until today, when anesthesiology has become a specialty that surgeons of all genres all over the globe are—indispensably—dependent on. Ether and chloroform suddenly made operations that had previously been impossible possible. More intricate, and delicate, repairs could be attempted because the patient was laying still and not screaming or writhing in pain. Nonetheless, as experience shows with any new solution, other problems, predictably, develop. Originally ether was dripped onto a mask that the patient inhaled. There was no airway protection for the patient. Plus, ether is extremely flammable, and caused drowsiness, dizziness, nausea, eye and skin irritation, and vomiting (for the patient, anesthetist, nurses, and surgeon in the operating room, especially without a well-performing ventilation system). At the time, monitoring of the heart rate was accomplished using a stethoscope or manually palpating a pulse, as pinpointing a patient's blood pressure awaited the invention of the sphygmomanometer later in 1903. This medical 'workhorse' consists of an inflatable rubber cuff (wrapped around upper arm), which was connected to a column of mercury and a graduated scale, that allowed the determination of systolic and diastolic arterial blood pressure by gradually releasing (or inflating) the cuff's pressure.

Thrills of Medical Discoveries

In 1961, Dr. Oscar Barry worked for one year as an Orthopedic surgeon at the Princess Tsahai Memorial Hospital in Addis Ababa, Ethiopia. Barry summed up the shared thrills of medical discovery during this time by writing:

> Medicine and surgery in Ethiopia have that exciting quality of a largely uncharted sea, with one or two well-known beacons showing the established pattern of conventional ways, but detecting nothing of the currents and the rocky shoals which are so dangerous to the voyager. Ignorance of these hazards leads to complacency and a false sense of security, which, in the realm of medicine, it is the scientist's duty to indicate and to help eradicate [...] Too often in this country a disease has been hidden from the light of the sun, partly due to the rural nature of the population [...] and partly due to superstition [...] When the early symptoms and the signs of an acute attack of poliomyelitis are not observed and understood, it is natural that the subsequent paralysis and deformity should be interpreted only in terms which *savour* [support] superstition and a belief in occult power.[176p47]

In conclusion, the quest for medical discoveries has been a nonstop journey throughout human times. We strive continuously to achieve decreases in mortalities and morbidities, promote mental and physical states of well-being, expand our knowledge of the cause(s) of illnesses, transmission routes, progressions of disease, while creating innovative drug therapies, diagnostic tools, and more. Now that we have reviewed some of the major discoveries that shook the orthopedic world, we will now conduct an orderly investigation into what are the globally accepted and standardized "Back to the Basics" principals of fracture reduction, traction, and immobilization.

Chapter 6

BACK TO THE BASICS

According to the NIH, bone fracture healing is "an intricate and fluent regenerative process that aims at restoring the damaged bone to its pre-injury state and cellular composition."[177] A fracture, in its most basic form, is any breach/contravention in the bone's structural continuity, with (some) degree of injury to the adjacent soft tissues. Following the fracture, secondary healing begins, which consists of four steps (with overlaps): hematoma formation (begins right after the fracture); granulation tissue formation (takes place within two weeks, providing provisional stability); bony callus formation (or if bone fragments are not in contact, a soft bridging callus forms), and finally, bone remodeling, that continues for months or even years after clinical union.[177] However, there are a vast assortment of fracture types, including: open/compound (breaks through skin surface); closed/simple (does not break through skin surface); stable; unstable; transverse (broken across the bone); oblique (angled fracture); spiral (twisting fracture); comminuted (many broken pieces); greenstick (bone bends on one side/breaks on the other, primarily pediatric patients); simple (one break); and complicated (surrounding damage to blood vessels, etc.). Despite these differences, some basic physiological principles in reduction and immobilization traverse across the (vast) majority of limb fractures. So, in order to proceed in an orderly investigation, it is necessary to organize our inquiry via the following (general) principals of reduction and immobilization, which include, but are not limited to the following: the importance of circulatory status of the injured extremity; the importance of healthy skin coverage to promote healing and prevent infection; the maintenance and restoration of proper form and function; internal fixation; traction for immobilization; proper reduction; complications (and how to avoid them), as well the use of imaging technologies.

When considering the fractures of extremities, it is fundamental to consider that our extremities are what we utilize the most in our interactions within our environment(s). Humans' lower extremities (legs, knees, ankle, and foot) allow humans a bipedal gait, standing, and many forms of movement, whereas upper extremities (arm, forearm, and hand) are primarily used for climbing, lifting, and manipulating objects. If you fracture or sprain in your dominant arm (especially those that include wrist and/or elbow immobilizations)—simple tasks like eating, writing, working, and even buttoning your shirt can become awkward, if not impossible. If you suffer an acute injury to a lower extremity, your gait (as well as short and long mobility) can be instantaneously affected. Many of the time-worn principles of fracture management have been known and taught for centuries in Western medicine. Certain principles—such as the critical activities of circulation—moving blood, bringing oxygen and nutrients, and removing waste—were not fully understood until the discovery of circulation of the blood in the 1600s.[177] The treatment of fractures, inextricably in many ways, progressed along with the advancement of warfare modalities.

Evidence-based principles involved in the treatment of fractures involve assessing any other injuries, stopping bleeding, immobilizing wounded extremities, recognizing physiological deformities, attempting to restore proper form and function, and ensuring good circulation. While it is easy to be distracted by an injured extremity that exhibits acute external bleeding and gross deformities, you can skip over (less visually obvious) life-threatening internal issues (such as spinal injuries and internal bleeding). However, after all life-threatening injuries have been addressed (like a ruptured spleen or neck fracture), definitive fracture diagnosis and treatment can be initiated.

The ABCs of ATLS

In Advanced Trauma Life Support (ATLS®), care of the trauma patient is divided into the following three stages: primary survey with resuscitation; secondary survey (a more complete corporal examination plus laboratory tests and X-rays/CT scans to clearly identify injuries and develop treatment priorities); and finally, definitive care. All 'Primary Surveys' are based on the mnemonic "A-B-C-D-E", which stands for A = Airway; B = Breathing; C = Circulation; D = Disability; E = Expose/Environmental control, according to the American College of Surgeons.[178]

As you perform the ATLS's Primary Survey, you immediately attend to the care of any acute issues—as they are discovered. For instance, if a patient has an airway injury/blockage/problem, you attend to that breathing issue straightaway when it is found, etc. Assessment of circulation includes checking vital signs, identifying and initiating treatment for shock (if necessary), and stopping bleeding. The treatment of shock may be initiated by administering IV crystalloid fluid (normal saline which is 0.9% sodium chloride, or Lactated_ Ringers solution), however, since most shock in the trauma setting is due to acute

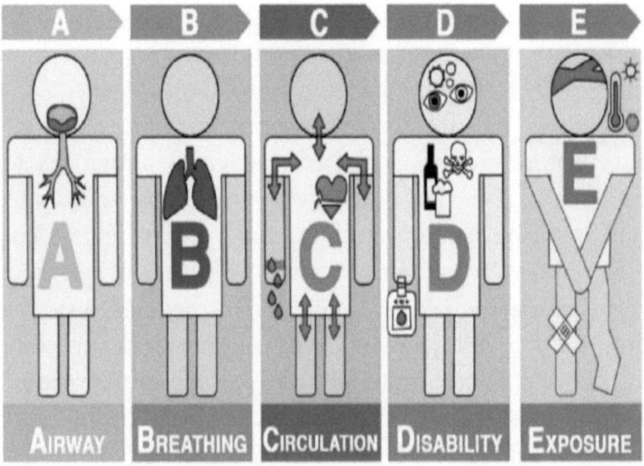

Figure 6.1 The latest ATLS® guidelines simplifying the use of their well-known 'A-B-C-D-E' mnemonic. Source: TargetOrtho.com, 2025.

blood loss, early blood replacement efforts can prove critical. The 'D' in A-B-C-D-E stands for disability, an assessment that involves identifying neurological deficits as well as deformities of extremities. Finally, the "E = Expose" orders the complete head-to-toe unclothed examination of the patient in order to see any (previously) hidden (clothed) injuries. This includes examining the back which may require 'log-rolling' a patient in order to prevent spinal injuries. Once this evaluation is done, cover the patient up and prevent hypothermia. The overriding purpose of this US-based approach is to identify critical life threats and address them before moving on to address other, perhaps more distracting, problems. According to Dr. Flowers, the 'team approach' is paramount so that timely and simultaneous treatment is undertaken: While the physician assesses patient, other team members can start IVs, draw blood samples for trauma lab testing, hold compression on bleeding areas, etc.

Once the restoration of vital functions is addressed and completed, the Secondary Assessment is undertaken, which adds on adjunctive information such as lab results, X-rays findings, and CT scan analyses.[178] Wherein orthopedic injuries will be identified, and if not already completed, splints will be applied. It remains imperative to check (and re-check) injured extremities' neurovascular status before and after any splinting, immobilization, or casting procedures.

Two types of potentially life-threatening extremity injuries include major arterial hemorrhage, and severe crush injuries (potentially resulting in traumatic/physical compression rhabdomyolysis, a life-threatening condition that is secondary to a mechanical force/crush injury or prolonged immobilization). Limb-threatening injuries include: open fractures, joint injuries, and vascular injuries (including traumatic amputation, compartment syndrome, and neurologic injury due to fracture dislocation). Open fractures/dislocations by definition comprise injury to the skin and soft tissues that connect to the bone/joint fracture. These open wounds result in exposure(s) of the fracture to contaminating dirt and bacteria—a high risk for infection. Whereas closed fractures can be treated with simple splinting or a closed reduction and splinting; open fractures always need surgical debridement in order to wash out any possible contaminants, plus a prophylaxis antibiotic regimen (to prevent osteomyelitis). Sometimes subsequent surgeries (including bone grafting, further debridement, bone regeneration substitutes, etc.) are required to achieve proper alignment, stabilization, and healing.

Subsequent immobilization techniques are then needed to re-align injuries (as close to proper anatomical position as possible) and maintain circulation so that healing can take place. The proper (or improper) immobilization techniques can positively (or negatively) affect the neurovascular status of the extremity. As an example, if a splint or cast or bandage is constricting blood flow to a patient's leg, this will eventually compromise the healthy circulation to the leg. In the illustrious words of Dr. AT Still: "The rule of the artery is supreme."[179] What AT Still taught his medical school students was that when blood and lymphatics flow freely, tissues can perform their physiological functions without impedance, however, when fluid flow is obstructed following injury, the tissues tighten and compress, resulting in localized under-perfusion, according to Hertford Osteopaths.[179]

Whenever there is a fracture dislocation, the urgency of its reduction depends on the neurovascular status of the extremity. Loss of nerve function or pulses in an extremity is a limb-threatening obstruction, so time is of the essence to restore proper alignment (and hopefully) restore neurovascular status of the extremity.

Precepts of Nonoperative Fracture Care—No Matter Where

When discussing fracture care from an orthopedic point of view, the predominance of fracture type is the fracture(s) of the upper and lower extremities. Additional fractures (such as rib, pelvic, and spinal cord fractures) are not really considered within the specialized purview of orthopedics—although they form a critical component in the Circle of Trauma. There are also any number of innumerable (and less discernable or observable upon physical examination) systemic factors at play during the time that a fracture is (or is not) healing. Some of the underlying issues that can affect proper healing of a fracture, include obesity, smoking, malnutrition, anemia, drinking large quantities of alcohol, endocrine conditions (diabetes), use of steroids (and other medications and/or illicit drugs), and old age. It is significant to note that the elderly population (physiologically) have a decreased ability to heal fractures when compared to younger populations. According to Meesters et al. (2018), the reason(s) why aging influences healing is due to an inherent weakness in the aged body's immune response coupled with an increase in systemic pro-inflammatory status.[180] While people living in a general population have a 1 in 100 chance (per year) to break a bone—the aged live with a 13%–50% risk of suffering an osteoporotic fracture.[180] With populations living longer than ever before, the observed global shift in proactive lifestyles in the older population will lead to people remaining more active until a higher age, increasing the population's potential fracture episodes.

In fact, the very latest state-of-the-art research published in *Scientific American* magazine in March of 2025, Denworth reported that a more active (as opposed to full immobilization) postoperative approach to fractures, especially of weight-bearing limbs, brings about a quicker recovery.[181] As a medical community, we were already aware that bedridden fracture patients were prone to blood clots, pneumonia, and muscle loss; but these new controlled trails are steering us to faster and less-risky outcomes. So, even today, our bone-healing beliefs and medical orthopedic constructs are ever-evolving as our knowledge morphs into today's 'Best Practices'. In Chapter 7, we will review the 'next steps' after appropriate ABCDE steps, including possible 'primary' complications and pre-/post-splinting concerns—such as circulation, capillary refill, splinting, pain management, malnutrition, patient comorbidities (sickle cell anemia), etc.—as well as potential 'secondary' complications (DVT, compartment syndrome, malunion, nonunion, amputation, patella gigantism, etc.) that may occur, especially if patients have or are currently under the care of traditional bonesetters.

Chapter 7

CASUALTIES AND COMPLICATIONS IN FRACTURE MANAGEMENT

At its core, a bone's healing processes are, in fact, rather multifaceted and prolonged, occurring around 6–12 weeks. Many varying physiological activities take place, including inflammation (hematoma formation at fracture site); a soft callus 'bridge' is created from cartilage and fibrous tissue among the broken ends; then a hard callus helps strengthen the site; then the hard callus is 'remodeled' into bone, and so on. Then again, acute open/comminuted fractures can lead to infections, and oftentimes, delayed healing time. Plus, if the patient is elderly, takes certain medications, suffers from hypertension, diabetes, is malnourished and/or smokes cigarettes—the 'normal' healing time can be even more protracted and even stymied. All of these physiological variances and keen medical insights—not to mention imaging capacities and capabilities—must be brought to bear by the physician on behalf of the fracture patient. It is never enough to poke contaminated bone fragments into skin openings and tie swaths of used cloth around an (obviously) angulated limb. In particular, four reported risky traditional bonesetter praxes include a "lack of radiographic imaging to confirm reduction; cutting and puncturing of skin with unsterile tools; and rebreaking healed fractures."[61p61] Primary (or initial) complications that researchers and physicians have evinced from preliminary bonesetter care oftentimes involves poor management of circulation, lack of pain management, malnutrition, and patient comorbidities, which we will now discuss in more detail. (More complex, post-treatment complications will be debated later on in this chapter.)

Primary Complications

The following topics involve treatment complications that comprise potential limb-threatening and/or life-threatening issues that may or may not be recognized by an untrained individual.

Circulation issues

When considering the science of Orthopedics, it is important to realize certain types of orthopedic injuries cause an inherent threat to the proper circulation of the injured extremity. In the human body, nerves and arteries travel together, so when a patient suffers from an angulated fracture or dislocation, the nerve and arterial status of the limb can be compromised. Normally, reducing the extremity into a normal anatomic alignment will restore good circulation. In non-acute traumas, the reduction and restoration of the bone's proper alignment may be all that is needed. It is always recommended to check the circulatory status of an injured extremity before and after reduction. Penetrating injuries often need to be explored to assess any possible (visibly hidden) damage to the arteries of the injured extremity.

Consequently, circulatory status must remain a paramount concern when immobilizing the injured extremity. Acutely injured extremities are prone to swelling, which may continue for several days. Healthy, robust circulation is critical to the successful healing of orthopedic injuries. Injuries likely to cause compromise of the circulation to an injured part are significantly displaced and angulated fractures—especially those involving joints such as the elbow and knee. Even when some penetrating injuries (that upon initial assessment) retain a healthy pulse, can in fact, be suffering from critical underlying vascular damage.

Splint removal or 'Bi-Valving'

Swelling that is constricted (due to a tight cast or wrapping) may actually compromise the circulation to the extremity or different muscular compartments—causing necrosis (cellular death) of the tissue. This is called compartment syndrome (which will be discussed at length later in this chapter). The underlying tissue damage can be severe and cause extreme pain, disability, or even amputation. Truth be told, the solution could not be simpler—quickly release/relieve the pressure. In a technique called 'bi-valving', the cast is cut on one or two sides, creating a kind of 'hinged splint' (that is effortlessly opened or closed). Sometimes the removal or loosening of a splinting, casting, or bandaging material will relieve a compartment syndrome; but sometimes a fasciotomy (an incision through the skin and fascia of the acutely involved compartment) is required. This 'decompression' relieves the pressure, pain, and allows for (a postponed) closure of the wound once the swelling surrounding the fracture decreases.

Checking capillary refill

Sometimes a patient's arteries are severed or severely damaged by a fracture, which can lead to thrombosis, necrosis, gangrene, and even acute circulation obstruction. This can be catastrophic and lead to necrosis and dry gangrene (to the extremity distal to the injury). This bone is now incapable of healing, and the muscles and other soft-tissues will necrose—necessitating amputation (if appropriate circulation has not been restored in a timely manner).

Unequivocally, there are several very simple measures—like using a splint (initially) followed by a cast when the swelling goes down and leaving toes and fingers visible when splinting or bandaging—that allow healthcare providers to check the patient's capillary refill (thereby ensuring appendages is not discoloring and becoming necrotic). What is capillary refill? Capillary refill is an indicator of peripheral perfusion (assessing dehydration or circulatory issues), and can be very quickly tested on the fingers or toes of an injured extremity. All that is needed is to press on the nailbed (which will turn white), and then release the pressure, counting how long it takes for the nailbed to turn pink again. It should take less than 2 seconds, but if the capillary refill is delayed—it may be a sign of circulatory compromise or dehydration and should immediately be investigated. This uber-simple tool (that necessitates no equipment) should be taught as an indispensable cost-free task for bonesetters to perform. Furthermore, TBS should be taught to: check both patient's fingers (or) toes to compare capillary refill times; recognize that infants and older adults might take slightly longer (up to 4–5 seconds); and that cold temperatures can slow refill times for every patient.

Pain management

Through our shared human experience, it is an accepted mortal fact that orthopedic injuries, fractures, and dislocations can be extremely painful. Humane treatment of these injuries requires specified method(s) of alleviating some (or optimistically all) of the pain—with the type of treatment varying widely according to the local availability and affordability of medications, pregnancy status, age (pediatric vs. adult), potential side effects, drug interactions, as well as the injury's location, type of bodily insult (fracture, sprain, dislocation), the extent of affected soft tissues, etc. Western medicine has an extraordinary pharmacopeia of pharmaceutical medicines that are readily available for this purpose. From acetaminophen and aspirin—to locally available anesthetics, narcotics, and other medications for sedation and pain relief. Ill-advisedly, it is the bonesetters' oftentimes aggressive and repeated 'deep-tissue massaging' of a fracture site that (invariably) leads to significant (and unnecessary) pain and suffering for the patient.

Pain from a necrotizing soft tissue infection can prove almost unbearable for any patient. As the soft tissue dies a slow death (due to no circulation) several symptoms usually occur: the patient's pain level increases (rather than decreasing in the healing process) to excruciating levels; they begin to sweat, become confused in their mental thoughts, and report a fever (higher than 100.4°F or 38°C) and rapid heartbeat (>100 beats a minute); the 'site of pain' extends past fracture area; swelling and discoloration occur (red, blue, or blackened appearance); skin blisters or 'gas bubbles' develop; sepsis (blood stream infection); pus (smelly liquid discharge) drains from area; and the fracture site begins to feel 'prickly' (stinging), then numb. While the numbness of the fractured appendage may serve to offer some initial welcome relief (whereas general public beliefs hold that pain alleviation = healing) to the patient, however, the noted decrease in their pain sensation is actually due to total nerve loss/death. However, TBS patients should not be lulled into a false state of relief, as a necrotizing soft tissue infection can very quickly (and permanently) kill skin, muscle, soft tissues, and lead to kidney failure, amputations, and death.

Malnutrition

Malnutrition is a grossly underdiagnosed obstacle among hospitalized patients in LMICs—as approximately one-third of patients[182] may become malnourished during their stay, according to Lovesley et al. Critical care nutrition, nutrition support structure or services, and in-hospital professional dietitian-led diets are all extremely underdeveloped and (largely) marginalized healthcare program areas throughout sub-Saharan Africa. When the supply of healthcare providers, medicines, beds, laboratory testing, surgical instrumentation, ventilators, and other lifesaving supplies and equipment are in short supply—a patient's access to appropriate sodium-free or high-protein meals (rather understandably), are relegated to secondary concerns, at best. Then again, this may be the easiest, most affordable, and least-complicated key to unlocking the proverbial Best Practices in fracture healing within LMIC facilities and TBS centers. Poor nutrition or malnutrition prolongs ICU and hospital stays, increases utilization of resources, increases readmission rates, contributes to higher morbidity and mortality, increases the risk of infectious and noninfectious complications, worsens clinical outcomes, and impedes functional recovery.[182,183]

"Next to fracture-dependent factors such as large bone loss volumes and inadequate stabilization, the nutritional state of these patients is a major influential factor for the fracture repair process," according to Meesters et al.[180] At its core, malnutrition is the physical condition in which a person's food intake is either is unbalanced—too low, too high, or bereft of nutritional factors. Concomitant with malnourishment is a low body mass index (or BMI), a state which also is correlated with an increased fall risk (thereby increasing fracture risk and contributing to nonunions).[180] A high proportion of the patients developing delayed union or nonunion were reported to have metabolic compromise, especially of vitamin D. Calcium deficiency is another compromising factor of the bone union. Calcium deficiency can be secondary to gastrointestinal malabsorption or endocrinal problems such as secondary hyperparathyroidism, according to Meesters et al.[180] Plus, according to the same study, adults over 65 years are at a higher risk of malnutrition, and a poor nutritional state increases the risk for osteoporotic fractures.[180]

Malnutrition is a pervasive challenge in rural Africa. For optimal fracture healing, the patient's diet needs to be sufficient in Calcium, Vitamin D, protein, Vitamin C, Zinc, and Magnesium—deficiencies in any of these components can impede healing and lead to complications (including infection and nonunion). Interestingly, many sub-Saharan public hospitals offer negligible to no structured or standardized dietary guidance (restrictions or other), nutritional supplements, or meals. Family or friends are expected to bring in food for their kin, church members, or friends. Oftentimes, due to a lack of dietary knowledge or financial capabilities, foods and drink that are provided to the patient, prove suboptimal for the favorable healing of the fracture.

Malnutrition in ICUs in low- and middle-income countries is 65%–78% (about two times that of developed countries); malnutrition frequency among oncology and infectious disease groups is even higher, 90%–100%[183] in the African setting, according to Abdoola. While there are indissoluble nutritional margins in readymade nutritional products for nasogastric feeding, for example, the costs of these premade commercial products can prove astronomical to an LMIC's public hospital budget. The procurement of feeding pumps, enteral, and parenteral nutrition is rarely deemed a 'critical need' and moreover, is "seldom reimbursed through government health systems"[183] in sub-Saharan Africa (Abdoola 2025), therefore, improvised 'home-grown' formulation options most be utilized. This homemade tube-feeding preparation versions, however, can lack the sterility (which can introduce microbial contaminants), calories, protein, vitamins, minerals, water, consistency, and flow needed by the patient.[264] Yet, global notions of nutrition, malnutrition, and top-down nutritional anthropometry (which identifies abnormal body sizes and suboptimal diets) may serve to suppress and "depoliticize"[p926] the structural determinants and subjective experiences of hunger, and cannot always be well utilized in many of these rural sub-Saharan communities, according to Smith.[184]

Patient comorbidities and pre-existing conditions

Many other medical conditions can impact orthopedic injuries, their treatment(s), and/or surgeries. When a fracture patient suffers from a preexisting autoimmune disease (such as multiple sclerosis, myasthenia gravis, pernicious anemia, reactive or rheumatoid arthritis, lupus, and so on), these diseases can actively suppress the patient's healing mechanisms, making them more prone to complications (like infections), and prolonging their recovery. Anemia (which could be the result of malnutrition), as well as inherited diseases such as sickle cell disease (SCD), will also delay healing. SCD is a hereditary hemoglobinopathy which predominantly affects people of African, Mediterranean, and Indian descent.[185] SCD is endemic to Africa, including all of the nations reported in this book. According to a 2006 study by de Gheldere et al., SCD is manifested via two primary mechanisms: 1) Hemolysis (rupture of red blood cells) leading to anemia, or 2) Vaso-occlusion (when sickled cells become entrapped in the microcirculation), causing tissue ischemia and damage in nearly all organs.[185] In fracture patients with SCD, they need to be closely monitored as they have increased risks of complications, like vaso-occlusive crisis, acute chest syndrome, osteonecrosis, and increased surgical mortality.[185] These patients should undergo 'peri-operative optimization' which may require hydration and/or transfusion(s), effective pain management, and the use of an incentive spirometer (to prevent atelectasis), which may assist to reduce the possibility of acute chest syndrome (a potentially fatal condition).

At this point, a cursory explanation of SCD genetics may prove beneficial. All humans have 23 pairs of chromosomes: one set from the father, the other set from the mother. All of the different characteristics that we have (like eye color, hair color, skin color, etc.) come from this, our genetic code. When considering the genetics of SCD, the gene for normal hemoglobin is dominant while the gene for SCD is recessive. What this means is that if a person has a normal HB gene and a SCD gene, the normal gene is expressed. These people are known to carry the 'Sickle Cell Trait'; they remain healthy personally, but can genetically pass SCD onto their children. Only when someone has both SCD genes is the recessive trait expressed, with SCD as the result (a.k.a. homozygous). A person can be homozygous for normal hemoglobin and will be normal. If two people (who are both heterozygous) have children, there is a 50% chance of producing heterozygous children (also sickle cell trait) and 5% chance of producing homozygous children, half of these (25%) will be normal and half (25%) will have SCD.[185] Interestingly, people who have sickle cell trait (are heterozygous for SCD; one normal hemoglobin gene and one recessive sickle cell gene), may have some inherent protection from some of the most serious forms of Malaria.[186]

Additionally, if a fracture patient has underlying hypertension or heart disease, the physiological stress of a serious orthopedic injury could lead to a heart attack or the development of congestive heart failure (CHF). Fracture patients who are smokers have increased risk of complications after orthopedic injuries and surgeries, including (but not limited to): pneumonia, heart attacks, wound infections, stroke, delayed healing, and increased risks of nonunion. Obesity also increases the risk of serious complications like wound infections, pneumonia, blood clots, and heart attacks. Sleep apnea (which often is found among obese patients) can also increases the risk of cardiac complications during recovery from a fracture surgery.

Post-treatment complications

The following topics involve more acute, posttreatment complications that comprise potential limb-threatening and/or life-threatening issues that cannot be diagnosed or successfully treated by a medically untrained individual, like a traditional bonesetter.

Infections

The challenges of performing surgery in LMICs, usually in a source-limited, less-than-ideal situation, undeniably increases the risk of infection, which, in turn, exacerbates the condition(s) of at-risk populations (the malnourished, immunocompromised, etc.). The routine absence of culture and sensitivity patient test results, the shortage of operating room time (for taking deep tissue samples), and the lack of isolation units (due to space shortages) are just a few examples of a surgeon's challenges working in an LMIC. However, even when patient's culture and sensitivity results are obtained, the necessary antimicrobial drugs may not be available or too expensive (especially in cases like a bone infection using long-term oral or IV medications).

What is quite confounding to many Western-trained physicians is how frequently African patients will leave the confines of a hospital with an acute open fracture case and seek medical infection care at an unsterile, ill-equipped outdoor bench of a village bonesetter. An open fracture is defined as a fracture in which the bony fragments have penetrated the skin, so the skin's natural barrier against outside germs is destroyed. Infections in 'closed fractures' (where the skin is intact), the risk of infection from contaminants may be nominal; however, in open fractures, it is substantial. The modern Western-care standard of practice of an open fracture is to immediately (within 24 hours) take patient into the operating room and complete a 'wash out' irrigation (debridement) using sterile isotonic saline (0.9% saline). Sometimes robust antibiotics and a 'delayed primary closure' is necessary, leaving the site open for a few days, so infected tissues and (missed) contaminants are not 'sutured in' (sealed into) to the limb.

M. Eshete's (2005) published article entitled: "The Prevention Of Traditional Bone Setter's Gangrene" revealed that out of 49 amputations (between 2001 and 2003) that had been performed in southern Ethiopia during two years, over half (25) were due to the onset of gangrene by circulation-constrictive TBS splints.[187] The rural hospital, Arba Minch, consists of 172 beds and provides the only surgical care option for the 1.5 million in the surrounding farming communities. The aim of this aforementioned study was to determine if it was possible to reduce this incidence of gangrene by offering one-day instructional courses to bonesetters. The courses were offered 10 times and a total of 112 traditional healers attended; additional two-day courses were given to 25 local leaders and health assistants, who also received training on the prudent care of fractures.[187] The same study's medical workers were given a supply of plaster, cotton padding, bandages, and written instructions (bonesetters were illiterate). After two years, the Eshete et al.'s (2005) study showed a marked reduction in amputations, from 49 (51% due to too tight splintage applied by a traditional bone setter), compared to 25 (28% due to too tight splintage); with only 7 (as opposed to 25) due to gangrene.[187] (For our gangrene-specific case studies, see Case #2—Solomon and Case#4—Daniel in Chapter 3.)

Gangrene

Gas gangrene (a.k.a. costridial myonecrosis) is usually caused by *Clostridium perfringens* bacteria, but other organisms (like Group A Streptococcus, *Staphylococcus aureus*, and *Vibrio vulnificus*) have been linked to the infection as well. They all can flourish at an injured site and swiftly rocket through the extremity, consuming muscle tissue and building gas and toxins, triggering both palpable crepitus and a rather noxious stench. Oftentimes, LMIC surgeons find themselves in a race against time—to quickly decide where the optimal surgical 'line of demarcation' (clear margin of infected vs. healthy tissue and perfusion) should fall in order to stop the spread—all the while balancing limb viability, blood supply, patient health, and prosthetic fit. Optimal rehabilitation for the amputee begins, whenever possible, prior to the surgical amputation, according to Admasu.

Another medically verified case study of gas gangrene (referred to by the author as 'traditional bonesetter's gangrene' was a "devastating complication arising from the practice of TBS with a prevalence of 4.29%," according to Luhur et al. (2021), citing that "most cases require amputation, which lead to permanent disability."[188] The three reporting physicians in the 2021 study (emergency, traumatology, and orthopedic specialists) note that a preexisting compartment syndrome is characterized by intense pain (usually out of proportion to the degree of injury) after the splinting. The patient's suffering and horrific pain was deemed "unrecognizable,"[188p4] but was readily dismissed by relatives, the bonesetter themselves, and community members as a "normal response" to the fracture and injured limb. In the aforementioned 2021 study, the three physicians go on to explain that the "tightness of the splint (along entire lower leg) created a "tourniquet effect," which led to a compartment syndrome, vascular compromise, ischemia, and finally, gas gangrene.[188p4] The globally peer-reviewed photographic, radiologic, and clinical evidence, according to Luhur et al., of the case study revealed:

> [...] a catastrophic presentation of the lower limb gangrene secondary to traditional bone setter's treatment. Traditional bone setter's gangrene is a significant contributor to amputations in many developing countries. The practice of scarification, massage with herbal concoctions and creams, and a tight splint may lead to infection, vascular compromise, compartment syndrome that may terminate in gangrene or death of the limb. This progressive limb-threatening infection emphasizing the importance of early recognition of compartment syndrome, adequate resuscitation or stabilization, and prompt and aggressive treatment.[188p4]

We would be remiss not to add an abbreviated note on antibiotic drug-resistance trends. Drug resistance can curb the uptake (absorption) of a drug, cause the drug to lose its efficacy (via detrimental genetic microbial modifications), affect a chemical 'inactivation' process against the drug, or completely reject the drug ('effluxion' of drug out of cell). A 2019 systemic review on bacterial infections and their antibiotic-resistance pattern(s) in Ethiopia demonstrated that the majority of isolates were resistant to routinely available commercial antibiotics.[189] Another systematic review and meta-analysis on gram-negative bacteria and their antibiotic-resistance patterns in patients with wound infections, similarly showed resistance to regular antibiotics used in Ethiopia.[190] This is a hurdle in many aspects. The current trend in the treatment of bone infections mainly focuses on a localized delivery system that increases the local concentration of antibiotics at the specific site of infection—while minimizing systemic side effects. Regrettably, many such modalities are not available in many LMIC hospitals due to their high costs.

Compartment syndrome

Symptoms of Compartment Syndrome include the 5 P's: 1) Pain out of proportion (greater or more extreme than expected) to the injury; 2) Pain with passive extension, or a stretching technique that uses an outside force in order to examine joint range and its quality of movement (example: pain with a passive straightening of fingers in a wrist/forearm injury); 3) Pallor (pale or discoloration of normal skin tone); 4) Paresthesia (tingling, burning, pricking/prickling, 'skin-crawling', itching, 'pins and needles', or a generalized numbness); and 5) Pulselessness (usually a late finding), explains Dr. Flowers.

While everyone would probably agree that a fracture will (in some way) be painful, however if after splinting these intense (out of proportion to the injury) symptoms occur, they should not be ignored. To check, the splint (or cast) and padding can be removed (as the acute swelling of the injury may have caused the cast or splint to be so tight that it is compromising the circulation of the muscles in the ortho-fascial compartment of the fracture). If not immediately resolved, it can cause the muscles in the compartment to atrophy—resulting in Volkmann's Ischemic Contracture (a deformity that causes permanent flexion of the hand, fingers, or wrist) or other deformity, such as 'wrist drop' or 'foot drop' (a gait abnormality that makes it difficult for patients to lift or move their forefoot and toes).

In such instances, all the splinting materials, padding, cast present need to be immediately cut off and removed. If removing the cast/splint does not improve the patient's condition, emergency surgery is required to preserve (any possible salvageable) normal function. Surgical management of compartment syndrome involves a fasciotomy (see page 208). The wound can be closed at a later time, after the inflammation has decreased. Fractures at high risk for compartment syndrome are fractures of the forearm as well as tib/fib fractures, extensive burns, fractures with a crush mechanism, or fractures subject to prolonged external pressure.

One approach to the prompt diagnosis of compartment syndrome involves measuring intra-compartmental pressure. Nonetheless, the most crucial factor is for the healthcare provider to scrutinize the aforementioned symptoms with a high index of suspicion. Other factors to consider in the differential diagnosis are a more proximal vascular injury. Any compromise to the circulation of an injured extremity is a time-sensitive case that needs urgent correction. The generally accepted 'principle based on practice' is: the longer circulation is compromised, the more likely the damage is to remain permanent.

When looking at an injured extremity, it's important to examine and/or X-ray the joint above and below the injury—so no other injuries are missed. Normally a partial splint with Plaster of Paris materials (or newer fiberglass splinting that is malleable but hardens on exposure to water and air) are initially utilized. The extremity will be wrapped with padding to prevent damage or ulceration of the skin from the hardened splint material, then the splinting material is cut to proper length, soaked in water to activate chemical hardening, applied while still malleable, and then wrapped with elastic support bandages. The splinting material usually hardens quickly—in just a few minutes. A sling can be fitted for upper-extremity injuries to ensure optimal patient comfort. A more rigid and fitted cast can be applied later (in a week or so) once the edema (inflammation from trapped excess fluids) has decreased.

The benefit of using newer types of splinting material (rather than an initial cast) is that the material allows for natural edema to occur while providing adequate immobilization. Usually this avoids the patient having compartment-like symptoms from a circumferential cast that does not allow for edema. Assuming adequate splinting and normal neurovascular status, as the fracture begins to heal, the swelling will reduce, and the cast will loosen.

Thrombophlebitis/deep vein thrombosis

Many times, orthopedic injuries require significant immobilization of extremities (especially with femoral, tibia, fibula, ankle, foot) fractures. Nevertheless, the use of long-term immobilization can lead to deep venous thrombosis (DVT blood clot formation in deep vein) which can cause increased pain and swelling, and may even embolize to the lungs (a life-threatening condition). Risk factors for the development of DVT include: familial/genetic predisposition; Factor V Leiden or Prothrombin G2021QA gene mutations; Protein S and C (vitamin K–dependent glycoproteins that have natural anti-coagulant properties); the rare Antithrombin III (ATIII) deficiency; and finally, other genetic factors like thrombophilia (hypercoagulability) and hemoglobinopathies (like sickle cell).[191] Acquired risk factors can include any number of variables, including: prior DVT; major trauma; surgery; pregnancy; malignancy; age (>65); immobilization for prolonged period; chronic inflammatory bowel, liver, or cardiovascular disease; obesity; smoking; certain drugs (hormonal therapies like birth control pills and Depo-Provera™ a long-acting, injectable birth control).[191]

Our focus on orthopedic injuries and bonesetters in this manuscript usually involves a trauma patient of some type. If there is a fracture (especially a lower extremity), it often needs to be fully immobilized. If surgery is warranted, you now have three major risk factors independent for thrombo-embolism (regardless of other considerations such as age, smoking, pregnancy, or inherited risks). Let us now briefly explore the pathophysiology of DVT more thoroughly. Whenever you have a fractured bone, there will be bleeding into the soft tissues from broken blood vessels in the bone and surrounding traumatized soft tissue. This blood that leaks out into the soft tissues causes bruising, and sometimes significant hematomas. However, this is not deep venous thrombosis. DVT involves the formation of a clot (or thrombus) in the lumen of a vein, which can cause obstruction to venous return and lead to increased swelling. Immobilization of the extremity (which is usually required with such an injury) allows stasis to occur in the venous system. In areas of stasis, where blood pools, clotting can occur, forming a thrombus. The thrombus itself can break away, travel through the ascending veins back to the heart where it travels through the right and left ventricles—but can become lodged and block the pulmonary arteries—causing a pulmonary embolus. A large pulmonary embolus can cause chest pain and is every bit as dangerous, and fatal, as a heart attack. With many major trauma patients, it is common modern-day Western care practice to put them on prophylactic blood thinning drugs (a.k.a. anticoagulants) to try to prevent the formation of DVT or a PE. Obviously, before blood thinners are used, the patient needs to be free of any sign of internal bleeding. Also, the patient will need to stop taking their prescribed blood thinners prior to invasive dental work, or surgery—and then restart the medication once the intervention is completed. The blood thinner Warfarin (Coumadin™) and Lovanox™, aspirin, nonsteroidal anti-inflammatories (NSAIDs), antiplatelet drugs, and new oral anticoagulants (NOACs) like Eliquis™, Xarelto™, Pradaxa™ need to be stopped—however, some supplements like Vitamin E, chondroitin, fish oil (omega fatty acids), glucosamine, and herbal remedies like dong quai, ginseng, ephedra, garlic, green tea, feverfew, ginkgo biloba, turmeric, and ginger should also be excluded from the patient's diet, according to Kaiser Permanente's (2025) study.[191]

The current diagnosis of a deep venous thrombosis is possible through the use of a venous doppler that uses sound waves to ascertain proper blood flow in the veins. If the venous doppler screening shows a DVT, treatment should be initiated immediately using an appropriate blood-thinning pharmaceutical. The medication should halt the ongoing formation of more thrombi, and allowing the body to eventually dissolve the clot using its natural mechanisms. Another approach can be surgical (a thrombectomy), or more advanced drugs that directly dissolve the clot. These more aggressive medical approaches, however, pose their own risks. Unfortunately, traditional bonesetters have neither the theoretical knowledge nor practical training to diagnose, treat, cure, or manage the patient's long-term risks associated with deep venous thrombosis.

Malunion or nonunion

The nonunion of fractures is defined as an 'incomplete healing' of a fracture where the bony cortices of the bone fragments don't connect adequately to support the function of the structure; whereas malunion is a fracture that 'heals with a deformity' (like angulation, rotation, or a joint surface that doesn't line up properly). In a malunion, patients may actually achieve bony healing, however the operational structure and physical function (like gait) is adversely affected by excessive angulation, rotation, improper joint alignment, and/or limb shortening (due to muscle contracture). Perhaps the most common structural cause for nonunion of fractures can largely be leveled at the 'tenuous blood supply' of particular bones that are characterized by a weak/fragile blood supply amid limited/compromised circulation. Certain bones, by their very composition and nature, comprise these (easily damaged) tenuous blood supply and demonstrate an increased fracture rate and risk when compared to other bones (tenuous examples are scaphoid, talus, tibia, and the 'head' of the femur).

Comminuted fractures with a large floating fragments, crush injuries, fractures (in which the fracture fragments are separated or poorly aligned where the healing powers of the body are unable to bridge the gap), and fractures that are poorly immobilized (allow movement at the fracture site) can all cause complications in healing. Each time movement of the fracture fragments occurs, healing that has started is disrupted. When excessive traction is applied by a bonesetter, heterotopic calcification (a.k.a. heterotopic ossification), or an abnormal formation of bone tissue in soft tissue, can occur (Alam et al.), and surgical excision can remove the unwanted growth(s).[82]

While unhealthy personal habits like smoking, drinking alcohol, and illegal drug abuse diminish and negatively interfere with effective bone healing, some prescribed pharmaceutical drugs have also been shown to adversely influence proper bone healing. These include the following categories: chemotherapy drugs (decrease callus formation); glucocorticoids or corticosteroids (may decrease bone mineralization); NSAIDs Nonsteroidal anti-inflammatory drugs; fluoroquinolone antibiotics (like ciprofloxacin or levofloxacin that inhibit cartilage regrowth); bisphosphonates (inhibit bone resorption/remodeling); and anticoagulants like warfarin and heparin (reduce bone mineral density).[192]

In modern orthopedics, femoral neck fractures are nearly always treated with surgery because of its high risk of nonunion. By using surgical fixation, the patient can be mobilized much more quickly (preventing the atrophy of the muscles supporting the hip that would invariably occur with 8 weeks of immobilization). Finally, such a prolonged immobilization sets the patient up for other complications such as pneumonia, deep venous thrombosis, or pulmonary embolism (PE). Clinically, when a patient presents with a hip fracture (usually after an elderly patient's fall), the involved leg will be shortened and externally rotated (when compared to the uninjured side), plus there will be significant pain with external rotation of the leg.

Patella gigantism

The knee, or patella, the largest sesamoid bone in the body, is an essential component of the extensor mechanism of the knee. On the superior end, the patella is attached to the *quadriceps femoris* muscle, one of the largest muscles in the body. On the lower end, it is connected to the infra-patellar ligament which is attached to the tibial plateau, thus achieving the extensor mechanism of the knee. When patellar fragments are separated, surgery is required, although some fractures do not disrupt the extensor mechanism. In regard to Harcourt and Echem's (2018) case study: "Patellar Gigantism Following Traditional Bonesetter Treatment"—an 18-year-old Nigerian male patient was diagnosed via X-rays with the closed patellar fracture, and was unable to extend his knee (so his extensor mechanism was disrupted).[195] For the following two years, the patient's knee was aggressively, crudely, and repeatedly harshly 'massaged' by a traditional bonesetter. When the patient returned to hospital (two years later), he remained unable to extend his knee and presented with massive "patellar gigantism" growth.[195] In this case, and so many others, if a close alignment (via immobilization) does not occur, the various fracture fragments will continue their repeated attempts to heal—even though the gap(s) may be insurmountable. Plus, due to the traditional bonesetter's detrimental physical manipulations and mistreatment of this patella fracture—the bone and surrounding tissue's healing processes were physically dislocated and disrupted by his injurious (and painful) 'massages' over and over. The patient in the case study was, ultimately, forced to undergo a patellectomy (removing a 0.5-kg "gross thickening of the knee joint capsule and synovium" plus "100 ml. of synovial fluid" was evacuated) and reconstruction of the extensor mechanism two years after the injury."[195p76]

Sprains and dislocations

Sprains and dislocations typically involve joints with the exception of fracture dislocations. Sprains are injuries to joints (in which the ligaments supporting a joint) are injured. Ankle and wrist sprains are both commonplace examples of this. Most ankle sprains occur with an inversion injury that injures ligaments on the lateral aspect of the ankle. These are the anterior and posterior talofibular ligaments and the calcaneofibular ligament. Many ankle sprains produce copious amounts of swelling, and may, in fact, show more even more swelling than a simple, nondisplaced fracture. However, when a patient presents with a wrist sprain—examine the patient's 'snuffbox' (the triangular depression located on the thumb side of the hand, explicitly on the radial, dorsal aspect) for tenderness—as this can point to a navicular fracture (one of the bones that is at a high risk for nonunion). If so, immobilization of the wrist and thumb is warranted. However, it can prove an almost impossible task to differentiate between a sprain or fracture without diagnostic imaging (X-ray, etc.).

The simplified treatment for ankle sprains is demonstrated via the well-known mnemonic device of "R-I-C-E": R= Rest (putting the joint at rest; no weight-bearing for some period of time); I = Ice (applying an ice pack to help reduce inflammation); C = Compression (applying a an elastic or compression dressing that supports ankle); and E = Elevate (keeping the limb elevated above the level of the heart to allow for the natural gravitational decrease in swelling). However, if traditional bonesetters or their patients use bathe the ankle in very hot water, or keep the foot 'hanging down' (not elevated), they can, in fact, exacerbate the limb's tenderness and swelling.

Ottawa ankle and foot rules

The simplified "Ottawa Ankle Rules" can assist TBS and LMIC healthcare providers to determine the need for radiographs in acute ankle injuries. This screening tool was developed around 1992 in Ottawa, Canada, and studies show it can reduce unwarranted imaging by 30%–40%.[196] There are five components to the ankle test (the Ottawa Foot Rules will be discussed later), and they are as follows: 1) Bony tenderness along distal 6 cm of the posterior edge of fibula or tip of lateral malleolus; 2) Bony tenderness along distal 6 cm of the posterior edge of tibia/tip of medial malleolus; 3) Bony tenderness at the base of the fifth metatarsal; 4) Bony tenderness at the navicular; and 5) An inability to bear weight both immediately after injury and for four steps during initial evaluation.[196] So, according to the test, ankle X-rays should only be required if: there is any pain in the malleolar zone; and (any one of the following) is found: a) Bone tenderness along the distal 6 cm of the posterior edge of the tibia or tip of the medial malleolus; or b) Bone tenderness along the distal 6 cm of the posterior edge of the fibula or tip of the lateral malleolus; or c) An inability to bear weight both immediately and in the emergency department for four steps.[196] Similarly, the Ottawa Foot Rules report that foot X-rays are indicated if: There is any pain in the midfoot zone; and (any one of the following): a) Bone tenderness at the base of the fifth metatarsal (for foot injuries); or b) Bone tenderness at the navicular bone (for foot injuries); or c) An inability to bear weight both immediately and in the emergency department for four steps.[196] Traditional bonesetters could be rather quickly and easily trained in use of capillary refill, the "R-I-C-E" mnemonic for ankle sprains, as well as the two Ottawa screening tools.

Even for seasoned healthcare providers, it is difficult to find a dislocation when a fracture is involved. Obviously, it is optimal to have an X-ray prior to any fracture reduction. The definitive case we can discuss is a dislocated shoulder, as the bony structure of the shoulder is not strong (when compared to the hip joint, for example). The body sacrifices bony stability to allow for the tremendous range of motion of the shoulder; whereas the hip is structurally very strong as it constantly supports the full body weight. Shoulder dislocations result in substantial disruptions of the shoulder's muscles (a.k.a. rotator cuff), with the preponderance located anterior/inferior. Historically, shoulder reduction techniques have been described for thousands of years—without many substantial modifications. However, what *has* changed is the ability to diagnose fractures vs. dislocations with X-rays, control pain, and attain muscle relaxation (via medication) for the reduction. At the outset, it is conceivable that bonesetters may have success reducing a shoulder; conversely, it also possible that bonesetters may cause more damage and pain to the patient. Any attempt to reduce these injuries (without any imaging diagnostics) poses significant risks of doing unnecessary harm to the trauma patient.

Multi-trauma patient

Much of what we have written about sprains and dislocations assumes an isolated injury that does not involve acute head, neck, or spinal injuries. Any patient with a loss of consciousness, blood originating from the ears, severe headache, or acute neck pain is immediately deemed a 'high risk' and needs to be taken to hospital for a more thorough evaluation. An example of a multi-trauma patient would be from a high-speed car accident, as they may have internal chest or abdominal injuries (in addition to their orthopedic injuries). Additionally, high-impact injuries can conceal unseen life-threatening lacerations, bruising, and internal organ ruptures.

While TBS may get a relatively good outcome when treating simple injuries such as sprains or dislocations, the outcome for complicated injuries is extremely poor, which is the chief source of grievances from LMIC Orthopedic surgeons. Oftentimes, the TBS practitioner's homemade 'medicine'—a veritable potpourri of unregulated, imprecise, and untested ingredients—burns, irritates, and scarifies the patient's skin (Panigrahi et al.).[197] The "enthusiastic application of tight splintage" (thought to help accomplish inflexible immobilization) "impairs vascularity."[197p29180] Many of the patients, who had visited a health facility initially, return weeks, or even months, later with acute complications like compartment syndrome, gangrene, malunion, and nonunion. Conversely, it is a rare occurrence for Western medical professionals to see any former TBS patients (who deem their TBS treatment as 'success') visiting health facilities later. In the subsequent chapter, we will take a global 'birds-eye view' of accessibility and affordability of orthopedic care, as well as per-capita healthcare expenditures by federal governments in our four selected African nations.

Chapter 8

CURRENT STATE(S) OF CARE

Before addressing any possible comparisons between the four aforementioned African nations, it is necessary to address the overriding issues of income gaps, Gross Domestic Product (GDP), median income, healthcare expenditures per capita, internationally standardized purchasing parity, etc. In a very abbreviated overview, inflation rates in 2022 between the four nations was 6.25% in Cameroon, 33.9% in Ethiopia, 31.26% in Ghana, and a crushing 193.4% in Zimbabwe; one year later in 2023, inflation was 7.38% in Cameroon, 30.2% in Ethiopia, 38% in Ghana, and a staggering 667.36% in Zimbabwe,[197] according to World Bank Open Data, 2025. By the end of 2023, Zimbabwe had the highest inflation rate globally, an alarming 667.36% change compared to the previous year, followed by Ghana (11th highest in the world at 37.53% change), and then Ethiopia (14th highest in the world at 30.22%).[198] The Ethiopian Birr and the Zimbabwean Dollar (now renamed "ZiG") have gone through a wide variety of macroeconomic and inflation-busting strategies, including the July 2024 launch of a floating 'free-market exchange rate' in Ethiopia (by August 7, the ETB saw a 100% devaluation in just 10 days), and on April 8, 2024, the introduction of the "world's newest currency" (ZiG)[199] by Zimbabwe, according to Reuters reporter Dawit Endeshaw in 2024. However, by the end of 2024, some inflation rates leveled out, with 4.5% in Cameroon, 17% in Ethiopia, 23% in Ghana, and a 55.3% average in Zimbabwe (per the introduction of a new currency Zim Gold (ZiG) being introduced on April 5, 2024).[197]

According to the World Bank, the definition of PPP GDP is gross domestic product "converted to international dollars using purchasing power parity rates" therefore, a single international dollar has the same "purchasing power over GDP as the U.S. dollar has in the United States."[197,212] Rossiter estimates that trauma costs global GDP approximately 3% per annum; conversely as trauma is disproportionately higher in LMICs (adversely affecting the working population in those LMICs), annual GDP losses due to trauma in an LMIC could be as massive as some 30%.[34] The WHO estimates that for every $1 spent on healthcare, a minimum of $10 of increased GDP is achieved

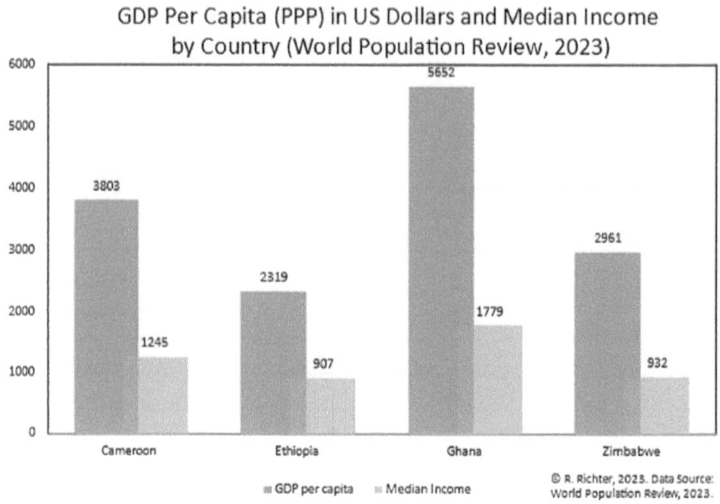

Figure 8.1. GDP Per Capita (PPP) in U.S. dollars and median income by country. Data Source: World Population Review, 2023.

in *any* country; whereas poor-quality TBS and healthcare can lead to work loss, reduced economic opportunities, inhibit educational attainment, and expend more costs, according to the WHO Global Health Observatory.[32] It is estimated that if the quality of trauma care in LMICs equaled that of high-income countries, then one-third of all trauma-related deaths would be prevented, according to the AO Alliance.[35] For good or bad, modern orthopedic treatment has progressed to very sophisticated, expensive, complex, and technology-oriented treatment options with minimal complications, and (predominantly) favorable outcomes.

Imaging Modalities in Ethiopia

According to Ethiopian Orthopedic Surgeon Ananya Admasu, the shortage of trained manpower is merely the 'tip of the iceberg' when it comes to working in Ethiopia. There is a limitation of physical resources including infrastructure, implants, and instrument sets; a lack of human resources (as other professions that closely work with the specialty are not growing comparably); plus, the absence of good administrative leadership in healthcare systems cause systemic challenges, Admasu explained. For example, she said, when a patient visits a regional hospital they typically (unless it is an emergency), will be given an appointment months later to be seen by a specialist. Admasu said her orthopedic patients are usually first screened by a GP/intern and then sent to the designated department (although mistakes often occur and the patient is sent to incorrect specialist), which translates into a circuitous duplication of the aforementioned process. The patients who have been correctly identified and categorized will then be seen by surgeons or trainees. A clinical diagnosis will be made and then sent for imaging. The routine '1st line' imaging is a plain X-ray. As there is usually only one (functioning) X-ray unit at Dr. Admasu's hospital in Gondar (serving hundreds of outpatient visitors per day, every day), many are kept waiting for days and weeks.

At its founding, back in 1995, the Ethiopian Society of Orthopedics and Trauma was established by orthopedic surgeons who had trained abroad. Over the following years, orthopedic training programs have been implemented in several regions throughout Ethiopia. The current number of practicing orthopedic surgeons is estimated to be around 150—serving over 112 million Ethiopians, according to Dr. Admasu. With the growth of training programs, the country has witnessed a significant improvement in orthopedic care, plus, Dr. Admasu claims the public's understanding of modern musculoskeletal care has progressed over the past few years.

Imaging (in the medical context) refers to different technologies using ionizing (X-rays, CT, Nuclear medicine) and non-ionizing radiation (MRI, ultrasound) to diagnose, monitor, or treat medical and surgical conditions. The technology of imaging has progressed immensely from artificial intelligence-guided MRI and CT scans to augmented reality in presurgical planning—thus, technological advancements and imaging mechanisms move hand-in-hand, correspondingly.

However, in resource-limited setups in LMICs, there is still a serious shortage of these expensive modalities. Any imaging sale (or charitable 'bargain') from global manufacturers are routinely only X-ray and ultrasound tech, so advanced imaging options are more concentrated in urban metro areas. A 2015–2016 survey of MRI availability in West Africa evidenced that 84 MRI functioning units served a combined population of 372,255,411 in the region, or approximately one single MRI machine per every 4½ million people, give or take.[201] Of these, 77.6% were low-field strength systems.[201] A more recent 2022 study analyzed 32 (or 59%) of African nations for MRI access, finding that less than one-third of countries had one MRI system, with the average of one MRI per million population.[193] Conversely, Libya, South Africa, and Egypt boast the highest per-capita MRI availabilities (followed by Morocco and Algeria), with private-sector clinic and hospitals dominating about two-thirds of all installed MRI systems.[193] The same aforementioned study revealed there were no African MRI physics societies; thereby allotting regional medical physics organizations the tasks of MRI education, research, unit repair, maintenance, upgrades, and training.[193] And sub-specialties, like interventional radiology services (such as radiotherapy) represent no exception to these sub-Saharan scarcity and accessibility challenges.

A study by Dereje et al. conducted in Ethiopia found that 9% (or 16 of the 178 surveyed women with cervical cancer) died while waiting for treatment.[194] The median wait time for treatment for the surviving 162 women was 137 days (IQR = 60–234 days), with 74.1% of women waiting for >60 days, 194 with tumor progression at 44.4%. When compared to women who began radiotherapy ≤60 days after diagnosis, tumor progression three times higher for those who began later, at 120–179 days (aOR =3.30, 95%CI: 1.18–9.27) and ≥180 days (aOR =3.06, 95%CI: 1.24–7.52).[194] This study directly reflected the countless lives that are being lost due to a lack of equitable access to life-saving radiological technologies.

Surgical Services

A systemic analysis of the Global Burden of Disease study 2019, showed in 2019 there were 11 countries where noncommunicable disease and injury disability-adjusted life-years (DALYs) constituted more than 50% of the disease burden. A study conducted in Ethiopia to assess the burden of injuries from 1990 to 2017, showed road traffic injuries, falls, self-harm, and interpersonal violence to be the leading causes of injuries.[203] Generally speaking, injuries tend to be very common in LMICs like Ethiopia, and globally most injuries tend to affect the young(er) and more fiscally valuable (career-productive) age groups—meaning that these are the populations that should be ensured skilled surgical care. Ethiopia, with a population of 112,000,000, has a 58%–76% working-age population (i.e., age 15–64).[203] With very limited access to modern trauma care, though, many Ethiopians forgo a hospital visit except in life-threatening cases or after all other conceivable low-cost interventions (herbal remedies, pharmacists, traditional bone setters, etc.) have proven unsuccessful.

The availability of surgical services in sub-Saharan LMICs, especially in underserved rural environs, can prove to be shockingly limited. The scant number of surgeons, the shortage of well-equipped and well-trained healthcare institutions, as well as the general public's largely "anti-surgery" stance—all combine to hamper Orthopedic medicine's bright future provision, potential, progress, and promise, according to Admasu. According to *The Economist* report for the AO Alliance, some 4.8 billion people worldwide have no timely access to surgical care, and 2 billion have no access to anesthesia for their surgical care.[35] In 2013 (in the Fako division of the southwest region of Cameroon), there were less than five operating rooms for every 100,000 people.[260] This means that elective procedures and emergency procedures constantly compete head-to-head for one of the few functioning operating rooms. In the same aforementioned study, some 2,460 surgical procedures were performed by 27.2 surgeons, (an average of) 1.3 gynecologists, and 0.3 anesthetists.[260] When we compare access to safe and painless surgical care globally, we see disparate alignments of privation cutting along deep-rooted fiscal divisions. Approximately 94% of populations living in LMICs suffer from a lack of proper surgical care, whereas only 15% of high-income populations live without surgical interventions.[35] On a more personal note, surgeons who work under distressing conditions, suffer from deep emotional upset, even PTSD. Sally Frampton, a medical historian at the University of Oxford, asked: "It was a really harrowing experience for both the patient and the surgeon. Can you imagine someone having to be forcibly held down while you operate upon them?"[171p1]

Infection Is the Devil Every Surgeon Fears

The challenges of performing surgery in such a resource-limited setup and under less-than-ideal circumstances dramatically increases the risks of infection, exacerbated by the (generally speaking) poor nutritional status, anemia, and other un-/under-treated co-morbidities (hypertension, diabetes, etc.). Even to this day, infection is the devil surgeons fear facing, said Admasu. Most of the time, empirical treatment is administered. Even in cases where culture and sensitivity results are obtained, some antimicrobial drugs are unavailable or too expensive (especially for the long duration that is required to treat bone infection via the oral or IV routes). A 2019 systemic review on bacterial infections and their antibiotic-resistance pattern in Ethiopia demonstrated that the majority of isolates were resistant to routinely available antibiotics.[236] According to the same study, resistance of *M. tuberculosis* for anti-tuberculosis drugs reached up to 32.6%; plus, *Neisseria Gonorrhea*, *S. typhimurium*, *S. virchow*, Group A Streptococci (GAS), and Group B Streptococci (GBS) were highly susceptible to most antibiotics; whereas methicillin-resistant *Staphylococcus aureus* (MRSA) was 'highly resistant' to most of the antibiotics (slightly increased susceptibility to Gentamicin).[236]

In an *Ethiopia Press* interview by Mulat in 2019, Dr. Biruk Lambisso, an Orthopedic surgeon, Associate Professor at Addis Ababa University-Black Lion Hospital, President of Ethiopian Society of Orthopedics & Traumatology, Head of Department of Orthopedics at School of Medicine/College of Health Science, Addis Ababa University, said the following:

> We have all the orthopedic problems the other world faces. The common ones are trauma, injuries, or accidents. Most of the fracture-orthopedic problems arise from traffic injuries, while the remaining causes are

construction falls following the booming of construction in every nook and cranny of the country, the raising of the country's economy, and other development issues. Natural disaster is also another cause in addition to emerging conflict, shootings, tribal conflicts, police conflicts, border conflicts and all that. Hence, in this big category, we have injuries which take 70% of our work [...] In a few years, we shall have a good number of orthopedic surgeons in Ethiopia. But in terms of service, some patients still opt for sub-standard or unscientific treatments. With time, increasing numbers of citizens prefer modern orthopedic care, and hence they are staying away from traditional medicine. I would say Ethiopia is very different at this moment in time. Our people should know the fact that modern health is better than unscientific and untested sub-standard ways of treatment. Therefore, they should be able to know the huge potential we have in relation to orthopedic practices in Ethiopia.[205]

Prehospital EMS Transport

Many orthopedic traumas tend to occur in isolation—and are (oftentimes) not viewed by other medical specialties and the nonmedical public as immediately life-threatening, *per se*, hence, it is these 'minor' (nonacute) injuries that are taken to local traditional bonesetters. In Ethiopia and many other LMICs, the rendering of rapid field assessments and timely patient interventions is practically nonexistent, especially in rural areas. For instance, in lieu of trained EMS transport, Ethiopian patients are forced to be carried by mule, or horse, or men on a homemade stretcher (like a wooden door) (called a '*Karezza*' in Amharic), or a three-wheeled '*bajaj*' motorbike (auto-rickshaw) transport. These low-cost, but laborious, transport options serve to discourage many patients and caregivers, as they would be forced to pay to travel long distances in order to access modern orthopedic care. The lucky few who do reach health centers or primary hospitals rarely have access to a trained orthopedic trauma surgeon, so they will, in turn, be referred to an urban hospital (which is even more far-removed from rural areas). Of the handful who successfully trek to be treated by an orthopedic surgeon, now face the stark reality of queuing for an extremely limited number of orthopedic surgeons and operating rooms. When the Operating Room is finally booked, the (singular) Orthopedic surgeon works with a general-surgery team (that lacks orthopedic trauma training). Finally, after patients complete their surgeries and are discharged—then the same worn and rutted groove of delayed appointments grinds on to repeat itself over and over again.

Through expert consensus, Knowlton et al. (2017) published a World Health Organization Bulletin stating the "minimum set of eight resource criteria" that indicated that the facility was able to provide emergency surgical services consistently (i.e., "always available" rather than "available sometimes" or "never available").[213] The three categories compiled eight resources considered 'essential for safe basic surgery' at a hospital. The equipment and supplies included consistent oxygen supply; essential medications (i.e. antibiotic, analgesic, inhaled or IV anesthetic, and IV fluids; functional pulse oximeter; and functional sterilizer); basic infrastructure included consistent electricity supply and a consistent supply of clean water; and personnel resources included an accredited anesthesia provider and accredited surgical provider. In Ethiopia, only seven of 19 studied hospitals (three district and four regional) met these basic surgical standards.[213] The most common resource gaps were related to personnel and supplies: twelve of the study hospitals had no accredited surgical providers, nine had no accredited anesthesia providers, seven had no functional pulse oximeters, and six routinely experienced shortages in essential medications.[213] So, if a hospital cannot provide patients a simple O_2 saturation reading from a common $10 Pulse Oximetry device, how can patients hope to undergo intricate procedures for severe conditions (like advanced cancers, major spinal deformities, or extensive reconstructions) that demand a bevy of highly skilled surgical teams (anesthesiologists, nursing, surgeons) as well as intensive postoperative care (ICU)?

Big-Ticket Orthopedic Instrumentation and Implants

Advancements in medicine go hand-in-hand with breakthroughs in robotics, compounding metallurgical sciences, Artificial Intelligence (AI), and medical technologies. The advancement, upgrades, and modifications of orthopedic-specific surgical instrumentation, implants, tables, pins, plates, and equipment (based on evidence, experience, and best practices) is an unending evolution. Especially in orthopedics (where implants are made of NASA-grade state-of-the-art metal alloys like cobalt-chromium or titanium or plastic polyethylene), there needs to be an equitable and corresponding investment in order to utilize these expert technologies. The tremendous monies that drive orthopedic surgical markets selling medical implants and instrumentation makes it impractical and fiscally unfeasible for best-treatment modalities to be delivered to LMICs like Ethiopia, Cameroon, Ghana, Zimbabwe, and many other countries. We can point to any number of reasons for these healthcare system deficits: a lack of prioritized (evidence-based) budgeting; bureaucratized/politicized corruption(s) concerning choices for purchases/

replacements; severely limited number of orthopedic residency LMIC programs, and a poor comprehension of orthopedic treatment complexities and day-to-day challenges by hospital administrators, legislators, and local/regional/national decision-makers.

Instrumentation

Shortages of proper specialized orthopedic surgical instrumentation in Cameroon, Ethiopia, Ghana, and Zimbabwe remain a huge impediment to such an equipment-intensive specialty like orthopedics. Globally, the costs of a hip replacement, spinal fusion, knee replacements, and fracture/dislocation of hip and femur, are deemed among the most expensive orthopedic surgeries worldwide. However, costs of any orthopedic surgery differ wildly, dependent upon overhead costs (equipment purchases/upgrades, staff salaries, and rent, just to name a few. With a very broad brushstroke, we view a range of orthopedic (elective) surgery costs from $4,652 in India to $40,000 in the United States—more specifically, about $3,700 USD for an arthroscopy in Poland, to an ACL repair surgery in the United States at $15,000, according to PlacidWay, a 'medical tourism' provider.[206] At this point in our study, it is beneficial to note that orthopedic procedures are classified into two categories: elective (scheduled in advance, such as joint replacements, spinal fusions, and arthroscopies), and nonelective (emergency/urgent fracture repairs, trauma surgeries, and amputations). According to FasterCapital in 2024, elective surgeries tend to have higher costs due to pre-operative testing, preparation, plus longer hospital stays and post-operative care; whereas elective surgeries have higher insurance reimbursement rates and lower complication rates.[207] In order to navigate the mazelike landscape of orthopedic surgical costs, digital medical travel marketplaces attempt to excise geographical limitations and patient–doctor conventions by offering less expensive healthcare options in 50 countries. On PlacidWay's website, the US-based agency advertises that Poland, India, Mexico, Italy, Moldova, and Turkey are the "cheapest and best countries for orthopedic surgery in the world where board-certified surgeons providing high-quality treatments in affordable prices" states the agency.[206]

When we seek to 'unpack' high orthopedic surgery costs, we see numerous factors at play, beginning with a specialized trauma/fracture surgical table costing between $70,000 and $200,000, according to Canada-based MediTek in 2024.[208] Like any builder, orthopedic instrumentation and implants are the tangible tools needed to reconstruct or replace damaged tissues, joints, and bones—including screws, plates, rods, nails, pins, wires, prostheses, grafts, etc. Advancements in these aforementioned tools can go a long way to reduce patients' pain, infection, inflammation, blood loss, and recovery time, as well as increase mobility, functionality, and overall durability. Technological advancements mean a perpetual cycle of novel best-in-class devices and implants—and well, these new devices and implants translate into more money for manufacturers, sales personnel, doctors, and hospitals. Case in point: the global orthopedic implant market size was valued at $48 billion USD in 2022, and is projected to reach around $72.08 billion USD by 2032, at a compound annual growth rate of 4.20% over the forecast period 2023–2032, according to Precedence Research in 2023.[242] The research organization notes that the market growth is due to a surge in orthopedic injuries; the huge geriatric population residing worldwide (falls and bone deterioration = low-trauma osteoporosis fractures and osteoarthritis); new robotics-assisted operative equipment; 3-D printing precision in structure for a particular joint/bone; and finally, the growing (global) acceptance of musculoskeletal devices. Nevertheless, many studies show that the prices of orthopedic implants are typically marked up 130%–140% across the value chain, with manufacturers and distributors taking 25%–30% of this hike, while hospitals glean anywhere between 40% and 50%.[209] For example, the same India-based report by Raghaven et al. showed margins on total knee systems at over 300%; while implants (on post-revision procedure) have an average trade margin over 4.5 times the published import price.[209] Across the board, though, we found that spinal fusions and hip replacements seem to take top billing for high-cost surgeries.

According to a 2017 IMS Health Study, the prices of orthopedic implants are typically marked up 130%–140% across the value chain with manufacturers and distributors each taking 25%–30% off any mark-ups, while hospitals procure anywhere between 40% and 50% of charges.[209] Even though orthopedic devices contribute under one-third of the total cost of many implant procedures—hospitals make the "highest margins in this business" reported the same aforementioned study. However, from the device manufacturer's perspective, as reported by Sterling Medical Device,[210] "Unraveling the High Costs Behind Medical Device Development" online statement from January 26, 2023, the overall price of a medical device includes these five main components: research and development (R&D), regulatory compliance, manufacturing, marketing and distribution, and profit margin. R&D alone includes processes such as: design and development, prototype development, component costs, testing for regulatory compliance, medical device clinical trial costs, and medical device administrative expenses. Sterling Medical Device also notes that next-gen devices such as "Class III devices and implantable devices that require extensive clinical trials and safety testing" oftentimes come with "a hefty price tag due to the expertise needed to develop a safe and reliable product."[210] In the United States, implanted orthopedic devices are considered Class III devices, which "usually sustain or support life, are implanted, or present potential unreasonable risk of illness or injury," with only 10% of medical devices in the United States comprising this category (pacemakers, implanted prosthetics, defibrillators, etc.).[211] Regulatory compliance processes for medical devices can involve undertaking lengthy and costly medical regulatory bodies guideline studies, performing clinical trials, device registration, study design, evaluation, and testing costs. Manufacturing these devices entails the creation of rather complex, highly detailed precision parts and advanced high-tech components. Today's current marketing and distribution of medical devices costs comprise not only advertising and distribution, but also compliance with (sometimes numerous) international regulatory requirements. Profit margins, of course, vary widely across the globe, though revenues are fundamentally based on the cost of product development, sales volume, and current competition in the marketplace.

State of Integration?

Based on several collaborative initiatives, it seems as though many traditional healers are, in fact, willing to incorporate standards and processes of Western medicine. For instance, in Zimbabwe, following a massive government campaign to end practices that could facilitate the spread of HIV, healers condemned using a razor blade, needed to cut the skin when medication must be rubbed into the flesh, on more than one person.[214] In Nigeria, Onyemaechi et al. (2020) conducted formal training sessions between TBS and orthopedic surgeons.[68]

In Ghana, authorities and practitioners have already actively considered the idea of integrating traditional medicine and healing into the public health sector. A study by Komla Tsey entitled: "Traditional Medicine in Contemporary Ghana: A Public Policy Analysis, Social Science Medicine" offers some insights from a public policy perspective on the transition of traditional medicine to future generations, the possibility of teaching traditional medical practice in formal academic settings (universities and medical schools), and how efforts to control the quality of herbal preparations (via biomedical research) will dramatically alter their costs (thereby undermining ease of access normally associated with traditional medicine).[215] Tsey offered that "there is very little attempt, however, to understand the contexts in which the knowledge and practice of traditional medicine are currently reproduced, let alone the social, economic and cultural factors that determine consumer choices," and added that the "reproduction of the knowledge and practice of traditional medicine in contemporary Ghana" holds the key to "potential public health benefits accruing from better understanding of traditional African notions of illness causation and preventative health."[215p1065] Additionally, Ghana supported the Primary Health Training for Indigenous Healers (PRHETIH) project (1979–1983),[200] later renamed Healers of Ghana. Interestingly, Warren et al. noted that traditional healers deemed sessions as "one-way"; whereby sessions on herbs were the most well received, while those that "consisted primarily of advice or description" were least welcomed.[200] These, and other shared experiences, prompted many arguments and proposals on how to adapt academic teaching and lecturing mechanisms for conventional healers.

Trad-Healers as Public Health Workers

As the incidence of tuberculosis (TB) was skyrocketing up by 360% in the Hlabisa district of KwaZulu/Natal, South Africa (in the seven years prior to 1999), proactive actions by the healthcare community had to be taken.[77] Unlike some other more complex diseases, TB can, in fact, be easily cured if patients complete their treatment regimen (for inactive TB or active TB cases—anywhere from three, four, six, to nine months) to kill all the TB germs. In spite of this easy regimen, there tends to be a high drop-out rate (due to lengthy time period). One innovative partnership between medical and traditional healers (that was shown to reduce the spread of TB) trained community-based healers to supervise TB patients and record patient dosages (ensuring proper compliance). One of the 25 traditional healers who volunteered in the campaign, said: "We were also taught about the symptoms of TB, so that when we pick them up in any of our other patients, we can refer people for a test."[77p90] Jack Nyawuza added that: "This information added to what we learn in our training as healers."[77p90] From the healer's and patient's points of view represented in the study, it reads like a win–win scenario: On one hand, healers welcomed their newfound respect within the medical community due to their augmented training; On the other, patients were pampered with healer 'house calls' at their homes when they were too ill to travel to the clinic.[77] The results were quite remarkable. Overall, 89% of TB patients supervised by traditional healers completed treatment (compared to 67% with other volunteers), with mortalities rates dipping two-thirds lower.[77]

From an epidemiological standpoint, traditional healers can be exceptionally effective in checking on and supervising disease outbreaks. According to Yale School of Public Health medical anthropologists Groce and Reeve, there is a conspicuous absence in current modern plans for global reporting systems involving traditional (or non-Western trained healthcare providers), "who in communities worldwide are usually the first, and often the only, health specialists to see patients with new or reemerging diseases."[224p352]

Groce and Reeve go on to state that: "These local health specialists, called traditional healers" can play critical roles in the "early identification of new or reemerging diseases," plus "assist in coordinating responses to outbreaks and providing public health education at the local or regional levels."[224p352]

Best Practices in TBS Teamwork

As we stated in our Preface, we are highlighting three Africa-based investigations and TBS-integration initiatives for a more detailed discussion. Onuminya's 2006 Nigerian study using a circumscribed collection of (only) one type of (simple) fracture—40 tibial shaft breaks.[8] As an aside, Onuminya also utilized a 'control' group for a more robust scientific comparison, an important key to any proper medical investigation, and one that is rarely found in any globally published TBS treatment accounts.[8] This particular TBS study, in our opinion, sets a 'gold standard' for analogous tibia-to-tibia fracture (parallel) comparisons, and also due to control group usage in the scientific project. Again, the authors believe that traditional medicine continues to be maligned and/or discredited, not so much for any innate or irretrievable flaws, but for not following an academically robust pre-determined line of investigation, i.e., the scientific method.

The second integration, a professed 'trad-orthopedic' initiative was undertaken by the AO Alliance nonprofit in Ghana—the Traditional Bonesetter Training Program, whose goal is to prevent disabilities and complications stemming from traditional bonesetter treatments though fracture care education. AO Alliance, based in Switzerland, envisions that by 2030, the "practices and complications of TBS for musculoskeletal injuries will be reduced by 50 percent"[9p1] in sub-Saharan countries. Since 2021, the Traditional Bonesetter Training Program, led by Dr. Dominic Konadu-Yeboah, has trained hundreds of bonesetters in basic non-operative fracture management.[9] In June of 2024, two large regional hospitals, Tamale and Komfo Anokye Teaching Hospital (located in Tamale and Kumasi), reported a substantial 60% reduction in pediatric amputations (due to traditional bonesetter-related gangrene).[9] Dr. Paul Kofi, a board member of the Traditional Medicine Practice Council (TMPC) of Ghana, (regulatory body for traditional/alt medicine), expressed how AO had helped with the need to map, train, and register Ghanaian bonesetters.[9] Using several local data collectors, the AO Alliance mapped and recruited 197 TBS from the Ashanti, Northern, and Upper West regions.[9] Since its inception, there has been a marked uptick in hospital referrals by TBS, and a 57% reduction in bonesetter-related amputations.[9] According to Yussif Abudu Babia, a bonesetter from Gwollu. Darimani, "I decided to do this AO Alliance course to improve what I was doing [...] I would like to thank AO Alliance for the collaboration with the hospitals so that if there are complicated cases that we can't treat, we refer them to the hospitals for further treatment."[257,261] According to the Alliance, the program's success is due to the collaboration of surgeons, nurses, data collectors, the NGO, and the local bonesetters. One of the program's trained TBS was Philip Abadzivor, a bonesetter and member of the Volta Region traditional bonesetter association:

> We very much appreciate the training. Some bonesetters think they know the patient's problem, but they don't tackle it well. So, the surgeons are ready to help us and to treat the patients when we are not able to help them. When we went to the hospitals to see what the doctors do [as part of the training], we learned that there are some things we cannot do, and we wouldn't have known that without the AO Alliance. We wish for every person who claims to tend to bone fractures to come to this AO Alliance training to see that they can and cannot do. After all, we are all fighting for the patients' lives.[9p1]

The third, and final, "trad-orthopedic" initiative we found of notable value was from Hawassa, Ethiopia, where a group called BOne Setter Associated Disability (BOSAD) has been created to prevent musculoskeletal disability caused by TBS via eight tertiary hospitals, Ministry of Health, the Ethiopian Public Health Association, and the Ethiopian Society of Orthopedics and Traumatology (ESOT).[250] To date, BOSAD has launched printed materials in five Ethiopian languages, an online application, and a prehospital management package for school children—hoping to transfer and "de-centralize" musculoskeletal injury expertise into its more rural environs.[250] However, despite these and other efforts, researchers (like Birhan et al. 2011) reported in Addis Ababa, Ethiopia, that there was "no form of cooperation" and a "lack of motivation to collaborate and communicate" with modern healthcare service workers.[216]

Yet TBS, for the most part, are not officially recognized, certified, or standardized by national medical boards, NGOS, and/or government organizations in sub-Saharan Africa. They operate comfortably well outside the distinct parameters of formal health systems, without having to incur any civil or criminal/common-law penalties, liabilities, accountability, or provider responsibilities, freestanding from medical ethics oversight, government-granted patient rights, treatment regulations for quality, safety and fairness, (or even plain old) 'customary care' praxes. In other words, their lawless medical care is practiced, for all intents and purposes, with both immeasurable *immunity and impunity*.

We are reminded of an old German proverb, "*Das Kind mit dem Bade ausschütten*" ("Pour the baby out with the bath"), which rather amusingly illustrates the importance of not discarding something valuable along with something that is undesirable or unwanted. So, it is not the careless *eradication, but rather the cautious reformation and integration*, of traditional healers that can best befit patients, providers, and the public health. Nonetheless, leaving traditional healers relegated to the sidelines—unsupervised and autonomous—will continue to have serious consequences. Some patients, preferring the healers, may disregard their doctor's advice or take herbal medicines that could have dangerous interactions with pharmaceuticals. By working with these healers (rather than against them), doctors would be gaining influential allies who live, side by side, in the patient's own community.

Better Than What?

The notion that "in many communities, modern medicine is not perceived as better than traditional medicine" was expressed by indigenous Bono healers without the acceptance of the connotative arrogance embedded in 'modern' medicine.[224p351] In truth, the dubious cooperation between indigenous healers and Western medical practitioners may be thwarted (at its outset) as Orthodox biomedical systems are ubiquitous: symbiotic and intermingled with affluent political and socioeconomic spheres. Nakuma (1993) suggested two-tier medical systems,[219] while others understand that 'integration' and 'inclusion' mean seamlessly merging the disparate systems into a coherent unit, and "identifying areas where the traditions can best complement each other and establishing a working contact in such areas."[200] Conversely, Barrett et al. (2004) argues that the barriers to integration, are in fact "substantial" and the benefits are "unproven."[220] With that, we conclude our investigations into results or consequences of selected traditional sub-Saharan African bone-setting, and move into how we, as members of the scientific, medical, political, and academic communities, might begin to implement positive conversations and recommendations—all, again, with a single-minded focus on patient welfare.

What we will explore next is a veritable "How-To" guide on the steps to take in order to undertake a feasible, successful, and safe TBS program that can: reduce the fracture-care burden on orthodox providers; grow a shared database; safeguard endangered 'medicinal plants'; and reduce limb malunions, malformations and amputations, etc. The recommendations are not in exact chronological order, *per se* (some may be simultaneous or unnecessary, etc.), however, they are written in a distinctly progressive manner, so as to provide a rudimentary guide for societies that are interested in skillfully addressing safer, standardized, and more coordinated traditional bonesetter practices in their own communities.

Chapter 9

ON-THE-GROUND REALITIES AND RECOMMENDATIONS

While it is possible for the TBS to serve as the 'first point of contact' for primary care patients with simple fractures, TBS must be purposefully and methodically incorporated into their national system of healthcare's training and certification processes. The reality is that, without any significant changes, TBS will continue to find a place in fracture care—with or without the interjection of safe(er) orthodox Western orthopedic sciences and practitioners. As Barrett reported on 'alternative' practitioners as healers who:

> [...] described themselves as healers, employing attentiveness, touch, and love to increase self-awareness and strengthen the healing process, usually in chronic illness, often with pain. They affirmed goodwill and respect toward conventional medicine, calling for greater integration of conventional and complementary health care; however, they identified the major differences of conventional medicine and several formidable barriers. They displayed concern about accessibility issues in health care and stressed that attitudes and beliefs were often larger impediments to integration than were economic or scientific considerations.[220p259]

Truthfully, as Orthodox 'Western' providers, can we (ever) recall learning to how "employ attentiveness, touch, and love" to strengthen our patients who are in pain? Perhaps there is, in fact, much for (both) Orthodox and traditional healers to glean from one another. The holistic integration of TBS into an LMIC's healthcare system may have a number of positive effects, including, but not limited to: reducing the fracture care burden on orthopedic surgeons, hospitals, and EMS providers; growing a shared fracture-care knowledge data base; integrating (meaning the incorporation of TBS knowledge into modern healthcare and ensuring that it meets modern safety standards) of community healthcare providers; the national protection of endangered 'medicinal plants'; reducing the number of patients with limb malunions, malformations and amputations; and safeguarding the usage of certain specified or environmentally protected ethnobotanical plants by certified TBS members.

However, in order for this process to be feasible, successful, and sustainable, several critical steps must be implemented, including some of the following recommendations (which are listed in a quasi-chronological/concurrent order):

1. **Prioritize trauma care** in your healthcare system. Based on the World Bank Disease Project, provision of prehospital care is extremely cost-effective—as low as $7 per year life gained for combination systems using lay people and professional paramedics, compared to $922 for anti-retroviral medications for HIV infection (See: http://dcp-3.org/chapter/2586/implications-urgent-care-needs-health-systems).[243] As we had stated previously, musculoskeletal injuries in LMICs are at the "breaking point" all over the world (no pun intended). When 83% of the 4.6 million deaths are from injuries,[35] there's an overwhelming percentage of individuals who, presumably, may have suffered unnecessary fatalities due to a dearth of supplies and services. Richter et al (2023) study in Kumasi, Ghana, showed that road accidents (RTA) involving four or more patients ('Mass Casualty Incident') incurred fatalities at a rate 1.8 times higher than RTAs involving less than four patients.[42] According to the AO Alliance (2018), a well-organized trauma system can reduce mortality by a staggering 15%–20%.[35]

   As one example, in 2023, at the World Association of Disaster & Emergency Medicine (WADEM) in Killarney, Ireland, Richter et al. "Utilizing the 'A-E-M-S' Algorithm to Assess & Spatially Link EMS Resources in Road-Traffic Mass Casualty Incidents in Kumasi, Ghana" was introduced, using a functional, cost-effective, evidence-based algorithm that assessed, prepared, trained, mapped, and geospatially linked EMS needs to current emergency medical resources.[42] The "Assess-EOP-Map-Simulate"(A-E-M-S) algorithm, created specifically for Ghana, initiated the spatial networking of RTA 'hotspots' to existing trauma capabilities and surge capacities across eight metro-area hospitals and included a sustainable "Disaster Medicine" university-accredited course training of 255 nurses, doctors, and paramedics from 79 different medical facilities.[42] The aforementioned study also showed how the addition of piloted quadcopter drones into any MCI/RTA scene management promised to be a real 'game-changer' in EMS MCI response, in that it will allow for four chief provisions.[42] First, the on-scene transmission of photograph/video of high-acuity patient injuries to skilled EM physicians, thereby 'virtually augmenting' on-scene trauma

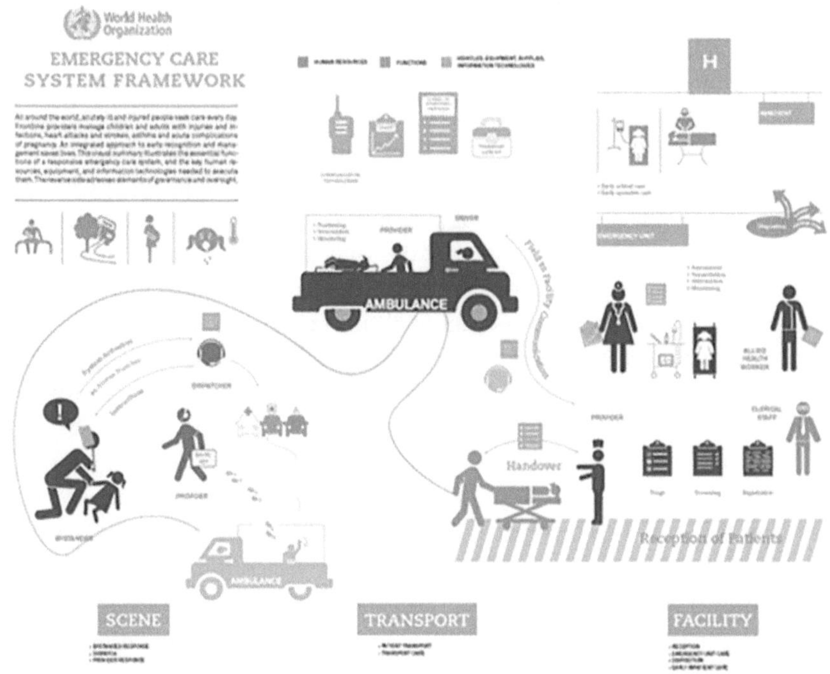

Figure 9.1. shows a visual representation of the WHO Emergency Care System Framework, designed to support policymakers wanting to assess (or strengthen) national emergency care systems, assess system capacity, set planning and funding priorities, and establish monitoring/evaluation strategies. The Framework shows emergency care functions at the scene of injury (or illness), during transport, and through to emergency/early inpatient care. This illustration also shows how ill and injured people who seek care every day are aided by frontline EMS providers. This visual summary succinctly illustrates the essential functions of a responsive emergency care system, and the key human resources, equipment, and information technologies needed to execute them. Countries can use this framework and WHO assessment tools to identify their gaps in care delivery and to create context-relevant priority action plans for system development. Source: WHO emergency care system framework, 2018.

triage skill(s) of on-scene EMTs. Improper on-scene triage by unskilled responders can have serious life-or-death consequences. Second, on-scene photo/video transmission of entire physical RTA/MCI accident scene to MD for skilled mechanism of injury (MOI) assessment. MOI—potential severity for wounding, fractures and internal organ damage (differences vary between 1) lateral/side motor vehicle collisions, or 2) rollovers, or 3) frontal impact collisions).[42] Third, on-scene photo/video transmission of kinetic energy forces. By understanding the "Kinetics of

Trauma," we can make reasonable predictions as to the kind, and even extent of injuries. EMTs and emergency physicians usually ask the same questions at an RTA—but now they have the advantage of being able to see the scene where injuries occurred (i.e., amount of vehicle damage, or distance of the patient's ejection from vehicle).[42] It should be noted that Kinetic Energy (KE) = ½ MV^2 (where "*k*" represents the kinetic energy, "*m*" denotes the mass of the object, and "*v*" represents its velocity). So, 'car-crash science' teaches us that the velocity at which an object strikes a person, rather than the object's mass, determines severity; hence, a car traveling twice as fast as another car will require four times the distance to stop. The forces in a car collision are quadrupled when the speeds are doubled, making a crash at 80 mph transfers four times the energy (to a human body, another car, tree, or wall) as a crash at, say, 40 mph.

As a fourth provision: real-time road access and traffic recognition for response vehicles. Drones can search for available routes in 1) inaccessible areas; 2) finding low(er)-traffic metro routes; 3) gridlocked areas blocking intersecting streets; and 4) flooding or mass riots/stampedes (collapsed or destroyed).[42] So, at MCI onset, EMTs on motorbikes drive out to scene, with UAV drone leading or following. Drones, like the DJI Phantom 4 Pro Plus (20 MP camera; remote controller/built-in screen; 30-minute flight time; 7-km. range; 4-direction automatic obstacle avoidance).[42] Our DJI drone shot 60 frames per second, flew at 72 kph, ran for ½ hour, and sent real-time images to a large-screen display in KATH's Emergency Room.[42] The published study showed that an early integrated approach to (on-scene) triage recognition and accurate on-scene patient management could save lives, particularly in Mass Casualty Incidents (MCIs).

2. The first step in the TBS-specific directive process is, of course, to first **identify the number of practicing TBS** in your community, their geographic distribution, and their level of known 'expertise' (such as years of work, local reputation, any injury specializations, sums of patients, size of practice, amount of assistants and/or trainees, numbers of fatalities, any long- or short-term patient disabilities, etc.).

   Using a national canvassing protocol, bonesetters should be federally mandated to answer queries on their service's effectiveness in successful patient outcomes, treatment failures, medical ethics, and sustainability concerns. A few recommended queries might include some of the following: What total (specific) community areas do you serve? How many patients have you treated? Do you keep any records of your patients? (If "yes" how and where are they kept.) What specific plants (and what parts: stems, roots, flowers) do you use in your remedies (and how you prepare: crush, dry, boil)? Have any patients become sick after taking oral remedies you gave them? Have any patients died under your care? After your treatment, are any of your patients unable to walk or use their fractured arms or hands?

3. **Substantial government participation** would be required as well as proactive participation by emergency physicians, orthopedic surgeons, national Emergency Medical Services, national medical boards, nurses, physical therapists, professional Orthopedic associations, professional global radiology organizations, NGOs, etc. The role of the physician would be to provide the necessary expertise and experience in directly training TBS without prejudice. Funding for TBS training sessions would be from government, NGOs, and public, as well as private-sector grants, etc.
4. Above all, the TBS community must be **sufficiently motivated** to participate in your proposed training program. This can be achieved by recognizing the participants as certified 'primary healthcare orthopods' or 'therapeutic bone technicians' or 'primary bone technicians' or 'trad-orthopedic technicians' (or some other culturally appropriate term) and instructing the general public in rural communities via radio announcements and telecasts to seek their services before enlisting a secondary or a tertiary institution for fracture treatment. This is a 'bottom-up' (or grassroots) approach that begins with local communities empowering themselves and their traditional healers to take charge of a safer and more 'sustainable' healthcare initiative within their community. Public accountability, responsibility, liability, and 'social ownership by the community members, bonesetters, and healthcare system is more than relevant—it's vital to its success. Even though the authors do not recommend that TBS be criticized publicly, a public awareness campaign should be undertaken that identifies the critical limitations between TBS' Protocols of Care (massage, finger and shoulder dislocations, possible simple reductions of closed fractures with X-rays, etc.) and modern healthcare facility-based Protocols of Care (open-fractures, surgical interventions, X-rays, etc.).
5. **Voluntary training** will need to be provided in the local language, as many of these TBS practitioners may be semi-literate or illiterate. Keep written materials to a bare minimum. Use colloquial (everyday language), photos, graphics, and simple illustrations that utilize only readily available supplies, local plants, and indigenous people examples. Whenever possible, use (clip art) imagery or photos to provide easy step-by-step instructions. One-on-one post-training surveys should be utilized to ensure that training session(s) meet pre-determined goals as well as local challenges and needs. TBS practitioners could be permitted and encouraged to attend as assistants in primary care trauma departments (as a part of the rural health scheme). Research supports the view(s) that many TBS practitioners would embrace

formal sector and/or hospital-based training. Yempabe et al. (2020) reported that an overwhelming 96.4% of their 28 interviewed Northern Ghanaian TBS expressed an interest in training courses, including recordkeeping (100%); pain management (85.7%), and management of open fractures and complications (82.1%).[62]

6. In accordance with WHO recommendations, teach bonesetters **basic hand hygiene, splinting, bandaging, and simple sterilization** commensurate with the available technology and local language(s)—this is a critical, mandatory, and 100% indispensable (and indisputable) 'starting point' to help suppress patient infection(s), Compartment Syndrome, etc. Low hygienic standards concerning any TBS's equipment, traditional remedy production, personal body hygiene, and treatment area/environment should never be allowed. One-on-one post-training surveys should be utilized to ensure that the training session(s) met (or exceeded) predetermined goals, as well as local challenges and needs.

   We can find approximately three comparatively successful examples of a TBS training programs in Ethiopia, Ghana, and Nigeria. One such example can be found in the Ashanti region of Ghana. About 157 TBS completed five fracture care units over a period of nine months (including pre-/post-assessments), followed by a formal questionnaire and checklist six months later. The modules (and pre-/post-assessment scoring) were: 1) Nature of bone and soft tissues (pre 3.62 ± 1.13; post 4.24 ± 0.93 = <0.0001*); 2) Fractures in children (pre 3.64 ± 1.06; post 4.38 ± 0.74 = <0.0001*); 3) Splinting and bandaging (pre 5.57 ± 1.79; post 8.04 ± 1.04 = <0.0001*); 4) Hand hygiene (pre 2.43 ± 0.64; post 2.42 ± 0.59 =0.8550); 5) Fracture complications (pre 2.01 ± 0.93; post 2.82 ± 0.45 = <0.0001*); 6) Pain management (pre 2.77 ± 0.93; post 3.61 ± 0.60 = <0.0001*); 7) Fracture healing (pre 6.68 ± 1.45; post 8.18 ± 1.31 = <0.0001*); 8) Record-keeping (pre 0.49 ± 0.50; post 0.73 ± 0.44 = 0.0284*) (those marked with * show $P < 0.05$, a statistically significant difference).[226] The comprehensive results of the program are as follows: there was an overall knowledge gain of 19.7% (67.2%–86.9%) in the pre-/post-assessments with notable improvements in record-keeping, hand hygiene, patient rehabilitation, and perhaps most notably, a jump in patient referrals to 37 over the half-year.[226]

7. **Record keeping** should be emphasized in all phases of TBS training so effective (and ineffective) treatment options, botanical usage, teaching methods, and implementation processes can be assessed and/or altered if needed. As seen in our (aforementioned) Recommendation #6, pre-/post-training surveys should be utilized to ensure that recordkeeping training meets and/or exceeds standardization criteria and local

healthcare provider needs. According to the National Records of Scotland government website, there are seven necessary principles to proper recordkeeping: Authentic (records are what they purport to be and who created them; added information must be signed and dated); Accurate (reflect the transactions that they document); Accessible (readily available); Complete (in content, context and structure); Comprehensive (document complete range); Compliant (complies with legislation, audit rules and other regulations); Effective (identified and linked to process(es); Secure (prevents unauthorized access, alteration, damage or removal).[227] As a rule, the (cost-free) sharing of data is not commonly widely recognized outside of scientific and academic Western 'spheres of influence' as a clever gesture, so the premise of 'knowledge sharing' should be patiently introduced and explained, as well as other ethical considerations, ownership, access restrictions, data storage and security, patient data protection, attribution, and fair use directives.

8. Seminars on the **prevention of complications** should be organized. These seminars should offer: small-group discussions, practical fracture-stabilization exercises (tailored to TBS usage of locally available tools modified to meet modern clinical standards), and visits to local-area teaching hospitals to expose the bonesetters to appropriate nonoperative methods of fracture treatment. Post-training surveys should be utilized to ensure that training session(s) met predetermined goals as well as local challenges and needs. There should be preapproved national 'therapeutic itinerary', if will, that outlines every single step that TBS are allowed and mandated to take for patient care. These set parameters, regulated by the Ministry of Health, that would prevent complications, must prove unyielding in their practical implementation and rigorous enforcement. Thereafter, any traditional bonesetter who is found working outside of his/her agreed-to protocols (such as pushing bone fragments back into an open fracture site) should be publicly identified in local media or radio, penalized (or jailed), and banned from any patient care in their district or region.
9. The **timely management** and referral of any complications in fracture management must be emphasized and understood by the entire TBS community. As necrosis is most commonly defined as 'irreversible cell death', gangrene refers to 'tissue death' due to some form of interrupted blood supply (like the too-tight splinting of a leg or forearm by TBS). From its very nature, gangrenous necrosis does not happen overnight—it is a lengthy and excruciating process. According to the NIH, necrotizing soft tissue infections may start as a lesion and progress to a skin discoloration and hemorrhagic bullae (fluid-filled blisters) "within 24 to 72 hours

of injury."[228p1] The aforementioned report noted that gas gangrene has a 25% trauma fatality rate—increasing to 100% with delayed or poor-quality treatment measures.[228] Therefore, it is imperative that TBS are taught to watch out for any warning signs of: fever, thin/shiny/hairless skin area, red, purple, or black skin in the fractured/splinted area (albeit is more difficult to notice on black/brown skin); swelling; loss of sensation, tingling, cold to the touch, or severe pain (after the initial fracture); sores or blisters (that bleed or release a foul-smelling pus/discharge). According to the NIH, the "early recognition" of gangrene "is essential to the success of the treatment strategies," as it is associated with a "high incidence of mortality, and in patients that survive, it can have a massive impact on the quality of life,"[232p1] especially with wide/disfiguring debridement(s). As examples, TBS can be taught to recognize reduced capillary refill, sprain and dislocation screening tools, fever, malaise, drainage, edema, paralysis, sensory loss, hemorrhagic bullae, severe pain (out of proportion to post-event injury), and loss of overlying hair.

10. TBS should '**brain dump**' **their quantitative data, experiences**, and/or qualitative data, when possible (including patient data, age, fracture, treatment methodologies afforded, any ingested medicines given, any topical medicines applied, malunion, outcome, possible disability, and function of limb, etc.). This data should begin the collection for research into the local usage of TBS and their outcomes for publication, public dissemination, an Android/iPhone mobile-device fracture care application, a shared web-enabled knowledge database, as well as future training seminars. While there are numerous reports that document the numbers of deaths inflicted by work-related/road-traffic accidents, disasters, and violence—few reflect the quantitative data collection of cost(s) involved in the care of the 10–5 'survivors' that occur with every single injury-related death, according to *The Economist*/AO Alliance Healthcare report from 2018.[35]
11. Interactive sessions between TBS and **local orthopedic surgeon(s)** should be made available—with focuses on human skeletal anatomy, reduction, immobility of the fracture site, as well as the identification of infections or life-/limb-threatening complications. There have been a few global efforts to 'combine the best of both worlds' by fusing Western-trained healthcare providers (orthopedic surgeons, physiotherapists, and nurses) with bonesetters. One such collaboration already in play since 2023 is *Stiching Shirati*, an Amsterdam, Netherlands-based NGO that supports the Mara region in Tanzania.[270] For two years, three bonesetters have developed treatment plans with local physicians (stressing sufficient pain management and X-rays diagnostics), whereby simple sprain, closed

fractures, and some dislocations are allotted to bonesetters, while complex cases are directed to the main hospital.

12. Establish regulatory mechanisms to evaluate, establish, document, and enforce a pre-determined **set of practice protocols for TBS** using national certification and/or licensure. Every healthcare professional works under very specific guidelines (outlining a prescribed course of action for clinical care), which are based on evidence and best practices, ensuring that care delivery is standardized and optimized according to the latest research and regulatory recommendations. Every single health profession works under a rigid (and inflexible) set of protocols. These formally agreed-upon protocols are to be a step-by-step 'roadmap' put into place to guide decision-making, decrease deviations in care, and minimize errors in the TBS practice. Each TBS should be mandated to sign/fingerprint an enforceable contract with an appointed government department or Ministry of Health (in their native language) that is legally binding in case of patient maiming/death, or other intentional hygiene or treatment infraction(s).
13. Undertake robust scientific studies on the verification, efficacy, and **safety protocols involved in phytochemical compounds** commonly used by TBS. High standards of quality control should be used to ensure the correct identification, accurate handling techniques, and (nontoxic) dosage(s) of plant segments remain safe for public consumption. Periods of review must be put into place to assess toxicity, side effects, and nontoxic dosages—as well as any complications from long-term use, usage during pregnancy, unwanted interactions with prescription drugs, etc. Once the studies have been completed, give all registered TBS a comprehensive list of "unsafe remedies," pointing out various indigenous toxins, overdose quantities of botanicals, unsafe herbal preparations, pregnancy warnings, common misuse(s), etc.

    A good example of such communications is the ZINATHA, or the Zimbabwe National Traditional Healers Association, based in Harare since 1980 with 55,000 registered traditional healers at 24 locations in Zimbabwe. According to the ZINATHA website, their organization boasts three services: a pharmacy (whereby registered herbalists certify herbs, so Zimbabweans do not need to "risk street-corner herbs"); consultations (by ZINATHA-registered healers); and coursework (unspecified certifications) (2025).[115]
14. **Address deforestation** and consider the fragile, at-risk and/or endangered status of local-area medicinal florae (including at-risk and endangered materials like sandalwood, white sage, white oak bark, goldenseal, bloodroot, blue and black cohosh, etc., and provide proven substitutes and/or enlist

the growth and purchase plants from ethical wildcrafters.[159] Determine the exact local gathering, drying (or not), extraction, maceration, and storage techniques of each endangered flower, seed, root, leaf, or berry—and whether it is a topically formulated medicine (applied to external parts of the body), as opposed to ingestion by mouth formula.

Already now, numerous studies are proving that rampant deforestation—propelled by agricultural expansion, mineral extraction, infrastructure development, commercial logging, and charcoal and biofuel production—throughout the African continent has led to higher herbalists' costs and plant inaccessibility, adversely affected individual livelihoods and national economies.[66,234] As we have already noted, 70%–80% of sub-Saharan African people use herbal medicine as their primary form of health care; even higher rates of 90% are reported in Ethiopia and Burundi.[66] Some researchers blame the ongoing exploitation of Africa's flora and fauna by 'developed countries' as the primary reason the continent has been unable to address their own usage and conservation.[229,233,236] Nevertheless, some communities have been documented that utilize a dual-system of herbal supplements and Western medicine in tandem.

According to Clark's 2023 report, Africa had a net annual forest loss of 3.94 million hectares from 2010 to 2020, ranking Africa's deforestation rate as the highest of any global region—decreasing plant biodiversity, as 33% of Africa's vegetation is "threatened by extinction," while another 1/3 is considered "rare."[66p1] Deforestation, according to Clark, "simultaneously presents two dangers to medicinal plants": as they are "cut down in the process of clearing vegetation", and "the habitats they grow in are fragmented, affecting plants' dispersal, species interactions, and resource availability."[66p1] Now, TBS practitioners can search many hours for a single plant they need, and never find certain plants at all anymore. This "increasing scarcity of medicinal plants" has hiked up herbalist's costs in Nigeria some 50%–100% (from 2018 to 2022).[66p1] Unfortunately, researchers are also reporting that herbal medical practitioners today have turned to 'more easily available' (although 'less effective') flowers, plants, and leaves for treating wounds and diseases—reducing the efficacy and cultural value(s) inherent in their treatments.[66,234]

Any losses in Africa's biodiversity, such as those caused by deforestation, can hamstring future global botanical discoveries of treatments for diseases and health problems.[230] As Clark skillfully summarizes in her 2023 report "The Impact of Deforestation on Medicinal Plant Species in Africa"[66]:

Taking action to prevent deforestation, protect plant resources, ensure adequate community access, and compensate for traditional knowledge used to create commercial drugs could guarantee that African medicinal plants can be used for both traditional medicine and global pharmaceutical research. In a world in which both disease and science are constantly evolving, it is necessary to ensure that the resources of the present remain accessible for future use and research.[pl]

15. **Nationally protected medicinal gardens** should be created as sanctuaries for rare and endangered plants, especially targeting those widely used for medicinal purposes. The all-too-rapid depletion of medicinal plants species must lead to calls for the widespread propagation of medicinal plants in-house or via 'patio' gardens. The rationale is that either form (wild or homegrown) contains similar biological ingredients, which may or may not always be the case considering soil, sunlight, and environ differentiations. Nonetheless, these medicinal plant gardens should decrease the need for wild harvesting, reduce gathering time and travel costs for healers, plus furnish a secure additional source of income. Special attention should be shown to local and regional festivals and rituals that utilize specific plants, as the collection, storage, and cultivation patterns remain pivotal factors. Communicative partnerships between plant gatherers, bonesetters, and plant growers can also discourage gatherers from over-harvesting unsustainably when they aren't able to sell their products in regular markets. One educational example of social media communications is found at Transjardins.org (Transgardens), a website that shows news feeds of educational gardens in France, South Africa, Eswatini, Lesotho, Senegal, and Burkino Faso, allowing children to share planting experiences and exchange gardening advice.[268]

Some modern-day examples of protected medicinal plants gardens within our four countries can be found at the: 1) South African National Biodiversity Institute (SANBI) which has 30+ medicinal plant species in Pretoria (www.sanbi.org)[152]; 2) Aburi botanical gardens in Ghana[127]; 3) Darwin Initiative for the Survival of Species in Ghana; 4) Shashemene Botanical Garden at the Ethiopian Biodiversity Institute (the "Wondo Genet" medicinal field gene bank conserves 320+ medicinal plant species in Oromia region)[221]; 5) Gullele Botanic Garden (GBG)[262] at Addis Ababa University (its medicinal garden was developed in collaboration with 24 key traditional healers), just to name a few. At GBG, a Memorandum of Understanding (MOU) was formalized, whereby healers share their knowledge on the use, preparation, and administration of medicinal plants and exchange plants grown in their garden; in turn, GBG propagates reasonable quantities of free medicinal plants.[233]

Legislators need to promote the national domestication of these targeted rare plants (for commercial production), plus promote 'alternatives' for propagating the wild populations of some plant species to "cater for specific needs of healers."[234pl] The wide promotion of the cultivation of medicinal plants in home gardens will, ultimately, assist in reducing pressure on medicinal plants of wild origin.

16. Standardize **mandatory label, dosage, and patient usage instruction(s)** on all herbal remedies sold to the public. From an ethical point of view, traditional healers and bonesetters are allowed consequence-free 'code of conduct' rein, as it were, to claim their metaphysical services and unidentified rip-off remedies are non-toxic 'medicines' with demonstrated efficacies. This rather '*lais·sez-faire*' Public Health attitude toward street vendors who peddle their mystery 'miracle concoctions' has led to the unchecked, uncensored, and rampant public abuse in the uses and sales of such unproven (and oftentimes unsafe) goods and services. The re-used roadside plastic water bottles filled with (any) variety of untold and uncontrolled herbs, grasses, mud, bark, leaves, and/or flowers, are ubiquitous in any and every sub-Saharan African streetside market and rural corner. Several researchers point to the 'explosion' of traditional/local therapies in different parts of Africa due to the lack of health care systems in rural areas forces local people to treat themselves, either by using medicinal plants or by buying high-cost medicine in the rural markets, or still further, going for cheap roadside medication, predisposing themselves to health dangers caused by the unknown source of these poor medications.[235] Again, it behooves each and every country to protect their citizens from financial ruin, bodily harm, and death from these cheats, who oftentimes knowingly, poach the public's pockets with their fraudulent 'miracle cures'.

The national standardization of herbal remedies for human consumption should address the following: usage; dosage; all ingredients and their sources (with the net % of contents); dietary information (% of protein, calcium, sodium, sugars, etc.); a summary of the essential scientific information (such as chemical profiling or macroscopic; and/or microscopic identification exams of ingredients) needed for the safe and effective use of the herbal remedy; prescribing information (such as contraindications for pediatric usage, pregnancy, etc.); any potential adverse reaction(s); any potential pharmaceutical drug interaction(s); storage and disposal information; name and place of business of the manufacturer, distributor, and/or packer with a domestic mailing address and/or telephone number; and concise, user-friendly container labeling in pre-approved national language(s). Vendors of herbal remedies should be required to operate at registered location(s), with permanent address(es), so they can be easily traced by clients, regulatory agencies, and law enforcement agents. The indiscriminate consumption of (potentially toxic/lethal) drugs without a prescription must be actively reduced and restricted.

As one successful example, the Traditional and Alternative Medicine Directorate in Ghana was formed in 1994 as a part of the Ministry of Health. The organization develops and maintains all "Traditional and Alternative Medicine" licenses, regulations, and standards within the subsector. Prior to this organization's efforts, these traditional practitioners were essentially unregulated.

Roadside vendors who refuse to adhere to safety requirements should be banned *tout de suite* from conducting any further public sales. The ban should also include the enforcement of punishment(s), including, but not limited to the following: fiscal fines, sanction(s) against seller from conducting any business within city or region, civil service labor duty hours, community service hours (with NGOs), restitution (pay the victim for harm), and imprisonment. The indiscriminate sale of (orally ingested) herbal remedies of unknown sources of substances predisposes the public to not only quasi-government-sanctioned fraud, but catastrophic health dangers, adverse drug reactions, waterborne infections, severe allergic reactions (anaphylactic shock), infant breastfeeding and pregnancy complications, irreversible liver damage, birth defects, and even death.

17. Initiate **local pharmaceutical and/or traditional medicine manufacture**. Drug discoveries (and appropriate patent filing) by state-owned manufacturers can bring in huge (and very secure) revenue streams. As an example, the largest share of patent filings in the pharmaceutical industry in Q3 2024 was in China with 33%, followed by the US (14%) and Japan (6%), according to Global Data (2024).[236] The biggest global exporters of pharmaceutical products are Ireland, Germany, China, Japan, and the United States, with some data reflecting the share of pharmaceutical exports for all of Africa at 0.2%.[236] According to the World Bank (2022) article entitled: "Developing countries have a path to creating their own pharmaceutical industries," LMICs should consider increasing their measure of national medicinal security by using new disruptive technologies (such as flow manufacturing) that require less inventory, use smaller-scale production facilities, have lower start-up costs, and are more automated.[237] Sub-Saharan countries can stop the 'bleed' of sending all of their citizen's hard-earned monies to another nation that manufactures commercially available drugs.

18. **Herbal-medicinal drug interactions** of locally utilized flora and fauna must immediately be assessed. Most traditional, complimentary, and alternative medicines (TCAMS) healers are unaware of interaction potential(s) of their products with pharmaceutical medications. The combining of drug therapies has proven invaluable in the treatment of many diseases; however, drug interactions can be complicated and even, at times, inconsistent. Therefore, it is imperative that licensed healthcare professionals assess latent risks of any additive, synergistic and/or antagonistic combinations on a case-by-case basis. The healers need to know what medications and herbal concoctions their patients are taking prior to any treatment. For instance, the long-term (more than 8 weeks) use of Echinacea has been reported to cause hepatotoxicity—liver damage/ toxicity caused by medications, chemicals, supplements, food additives, alcohol, etc.—and should not be used with anabolic steroids, amiodarone, methotrexate, or ketoconazole.[3] Non-steroidal anti-inflammatory drugs (NSAIDs) have been shown to 'negate' any benefit in the usage of feverfew for migraine headaches, plus feverfew, garlic, ginger, and ginseng have been reported to alter bleeding time, according to Fokunang et al.—and not be used concomitantly with warfarin sodium (salt form of warfarin, a coumarin, and vitamin K antagonist with anticoagulant activity, used by patients to prevent blood clots).[3] Ginseng (oftentimes an ingredient in herbal concoctions) studies have shown that the herb can cause headaches, tremors, and manic episodes in combination with phenelzine sulfate, and should not be used in combination with estrogen or corticosteroids, as reported by Fokunang et al.'s Cameroon study in 2011.[3]
19. TBS must be **formally incorporated into the National Health System via mediation**. Some form of (culturally appropriate) recognition of the certified TBS as genuine primary healthcare providers for first aid, simple dislocation(s) and (some) closed simple fracture bandaging and splinting prior to diagnostic X-rays. The reported antagonism between orthodox (Western) and unorthodox (traditional) practitioners may well be hyperbole, as both factions realize they must find ways to conform on behalf of the patient's economic and physical wellbeing. Nevertheless, this yawning and unplumbed chasm of mistrust must be (somehow) traversed.[217]

Clearly, the deep-rooted 'secrecy' aspects of African traditional medicine healers' care regimens—*perhaps the most unassailable (and controlling) means they wield*—will neither be sacrificed quickly nor easily. Biomedical practitioners (whether out of a lack of tolerance or acquiescence) will no doubt characterize this as a 'tacit confirmation' of its inherently fraudulent nature. Equally, biomedicine effectively condones for-profit care machinations through its facilities, intellectual property limits, market controls, lobbying efforts (amounting to $750,838,554 in 2024 in the United States alone), biased legislative voting (in 2024, the United States had 3,264 healthcare sector lobbyists).[266] Case in Point: Despite the obvious (and rather dubious) incentives for self-referral, US physician-owned hospitals can legally 'cherry pick' healthier and wealthier patients—by turning away patients who are uninsured or have complex medical needs, and/or offering only specific highly profitable specialties. So understandably, and rightfully, traditional bonesetters and healers view the interest of non-African providers as a profit-seeking rip-off—whereby the Westerners glean colossal profits and swindle the traditional healers, who are left disregarded, disrespected, and financially uncompensated.

In these cases, the authors urge the contesting parties to consider a third-party mediation, a process that utilizes a mutually selected 'third party' (an impartial/neutral person) to define problems, allow for equitable communications, avoid confrontation/ill will, negotiate their differences, and find the shared 'sweet spot' of common ground. During these meetings, all of the power lies strictly with the two parties, and not the mediator (who does not assess guilt or innocence, fairness or injustices), rather he/she has each side make concessions until a mutually amenable pact is reached. It behooves us to note that an attitude of superiority (from either side) will undermine trust and serve to quickly squelch any burgeoning collaboration effort.

20. **Physiotherapists** need to be included in the training program of TBS as they are instrumental in teaching the TBS some basic forms of post-trauma rehabilitation exercises for patients. Physiotherapists, according to Nigeria-based St. Joseph's Physiotherapy Clinic, focus on physical rehabilitation, employing "targeted exercises and therapies to restore mobility and functionality to the fractured bones," and that this is done with "evidence-based research, techniques and physical modalities such as ultrasound therapy, cryotherapy, heat therapy, shockwave therapy, electrotherapy etc."[245p1] Physiotherapy sessions, when conducted in a timely fashion by an accredited professional, can offer fracture patients a quicker return to full function, as well as a more efficacious rehab outcome.

As an example, in the United States, DPTs, or doctors of physical therapy (hold graduate-level first professional degree or doctorate degree for professional practice); physiotherapists (work with injured bodies and focus on pain management and rehabilitation); and physical trainers (who work with healthy bodies and focus on building muscle mass, fitness, and aesthetics) are all trained in the basics of human anatomy and physiology. For example, a physical therapist in the United States can train 7–8 years, and must earn a Doctor of Physical Therapy (DPT) degree, complete clinical rotations, and pass the National Physical Therapy Examination (NPTE). The length of most professional DPT programs is about three years and covers the study of biology, anatomy, cellular histology, physiology, exercise physiology, biomechanics, kinesiology, neuroscience, pharmacology, pathology, behavioral sciences, communication, ethics, management, finance, sociology, clinical reasoning, evidence-based practices, as well as cardiovascular, pulmonary, endocrine, metabolic, and musculoskeletal systems. Approximately two-thirds of the DPT curriculum are didactic instruction and lab study, with the remaining one-third dedicated to clinical education (an average of 22 weeks), according to the American Physical Therapy Association in 2025.[238]

Of course there are many schools of physiotherapy techniques, with each endorsing its own variation(s) of healing and exercise, but at its core physiotherapy includes: healing; encouraging weight-bearing movement; maintaining strength of weakened muscles; maintaining range of movement of the affected and surrounding joints; reducing pain; reducing swelling; returning to full function; returning strength and full range of movement to muscles and joints; and finally, optimizing the range of movement at the affected joint, as reported by Physio.co.uk in 2025.[222]

21. Create easy-to-use **Android/iPhone Fracture Care management algorithm application** (in simplified native language) whereby TBS would be able to easily follow a 'roadmap' of scenarios, such as: whether a fracture is open or closed; if trauma is most likely a dislocation or sprain or fracture; how to properly bandage specified appendage (nose, forearm, wrist, shoulder, femur, ankle, etc.) either for safe patient transport or treatment. See some current online examples of simple illustrations and/or photos that could be helpful in the TBS (or medical layperson's) assessment and treatment of various bone injuries.

When we view Figure 9.4, we see how Omololu distinctly separates the routes in her fracture care algorithm for TBS between 'closed' and 'open' fractures, and then again for 'displaced' or 'un-displaced' (or sometimes called "dislocated" or "non-dislocated").[265] When a fracture is displaced, the ends of the bone are out of their proper anatomical alignment, and the broken bone (or parts of the bone) need to be set back into alignment. As we have stated previously, the step(s) in which someone (manually or surgically) realigns (or 'reduces') the bone is extremely critical to the patient's recovery and successful outcome.

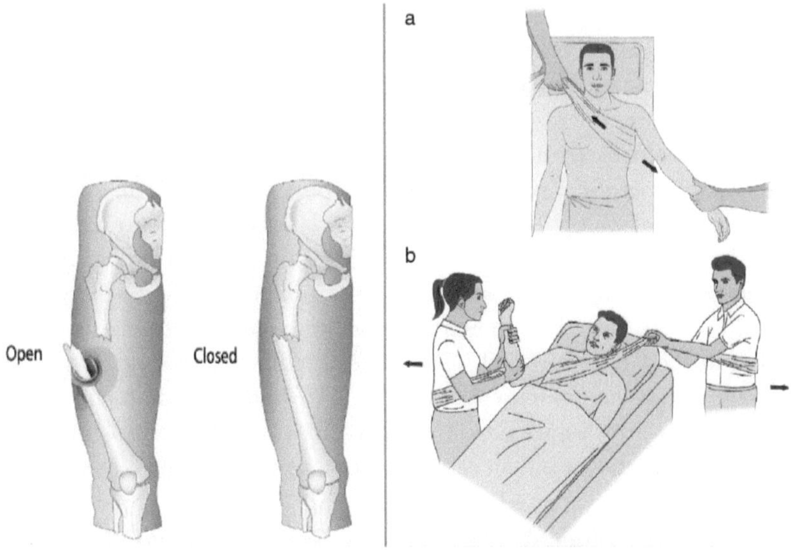

Figure 9.2 & 9.3. (L) A simplified diagram illustrating open vs. closed fractures (Source: Facty.com 2018). (R) Steps to reduce a Glenohumeral Joint dislocation (Source: Vinbaak et al, 2020).

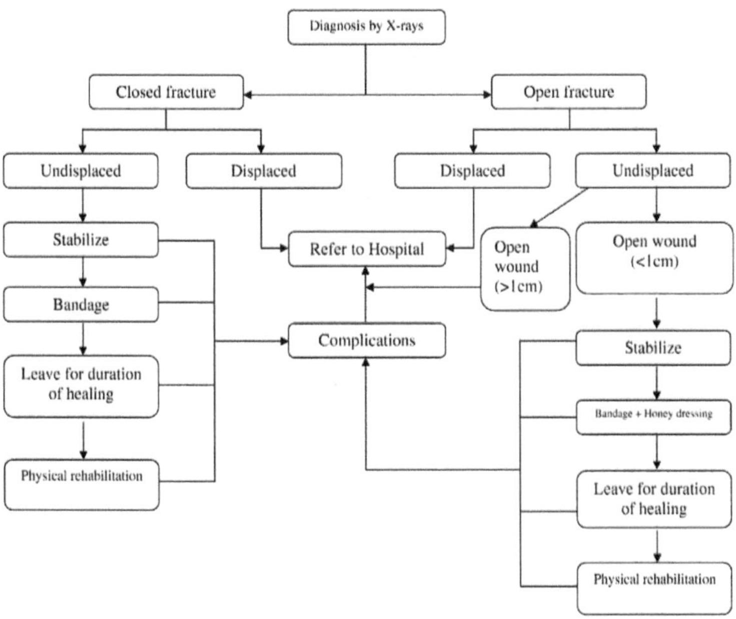

Figure 9.4. In 2008, Omololu[265] published a simplified TBS algorithm for the Nigerian region in: "The practice of traditional bone setting: Training algorithm". (Source: Omololu AB, 2008).

This multilingual Android/iPhone application could also allow user to send photos (and perhaps short videos of gait, rotational movement, etc.) to orthopedic professionals and receive (nonjudgmental) medical advice on patient treatment or physiotherapy. There are already thousands of simple fracture care algorithms available online, however, modifications as to ease-of-use, graphics, photographs, simplified language, and sociocultural aspects would need to be defined per each regional area of the country. Another simplified algorithm is found in Figure 9.5, A fracture-care algorithm under current online use by 60SecondMed, 2025.[202] The four "R's" shown in algorithm include Resuscitate, Reduce, Retain, and Rehab, which allows for a comprehensive approach from triage intake to outpatient outcome. We highly recommend using a comprehensive end-to-end (all-inclusive) like this algorithm, which allows for A-B-C-D-E assessment so that other wounds, internal bleeding, and/or fractures are not missed.

22. Create a **<u>web-based Q&A forum for your local TBS</u>** so the practitioners may ask questions, send photos, and receive medical assistance from medical professionals in their own (written or verbally recorded) native language. These Internet forums (a.k.a. message boards; WhatsApp group chats, etc.) offer cost-free online discussion sites where bonesetters, patients, physiotherapists, and orthopedic specialists could hold conversations in the form of posted messages (whereas chat rooms offer only short texts). These 'Q&A' conversations offer a virtual classroom for like-minded individuals, and their queries and responses are (commonly) temporarily archived, so others can view them as well.

    These mega-popular traditional forum sites include well-known industry giants—the likes of Reddit.com (1.6 billion users), Quora.

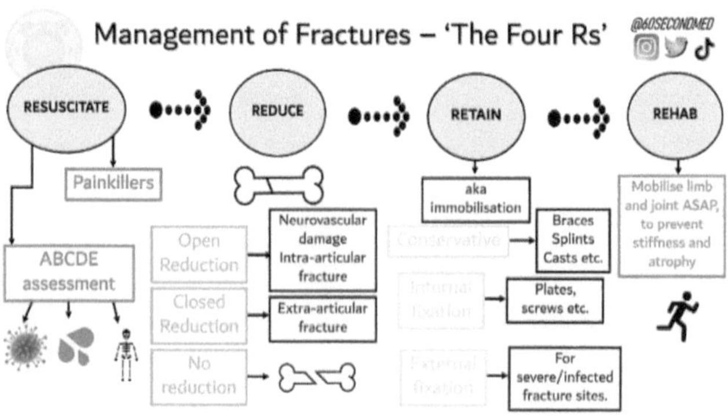

Figure 9.5. A fracture-care algorithm under current online use by 60SecondMed, 2025.[202]

com (500 million users), and Stackoverflow.com (274.4 million users), as of 2022, reports Rudzki.[239] Of course, not everyone is interested in fractures, bone-setting techniques, and orthopedic trauma care, so smaller specialized community-building tools like Discord and Slack or social media groups like Facebook can serve populations dedicated to one particular challenge. According to Rudzki (2022), a well-run online forum should show "straightforward and easily findable answers to specific questions," validate authors and areas of expertise, use name and surname of all posting authors, and place "high-quality answers" near the top of the page.[239pl] Especially due to the fact that people's healthcare, limbs, and lives would be placed "up for discussion"—unwavering professionalism and accountability of the site's content would remain paramount. Therefore, there should not be any 'unverified' responses from anonymous accounts allowed on these types of forums.

23. Eventually, all TBS should be required to take **biannual or annual training** in order to be certified to practice by the (responsible) government entities. Government-appointed medical personnel would carry out routine inspection of TBS practices and facilities in order to ensure the proper standards of health care are being met, and hopefully, exceeded. Training modules should include information previously addressed in Chapters 6–8.
24. Doing to burgeoning patient numbers, LMICs need to **increase orthopedic training opportunities** for surgical professionals (especially women and other marginalized groups) in order to improve access to Orthopedic instrumentation, surgical implants, and imaging modalities, as well as regulate the quality of hospital-based services. Recently, in 2020, there was an introduction of an online surgical instruction app by Bonesetter Solutions LLC in Ann Arbor Michigan, USA (httpsfako://detroitbonesetter.com).[240] This online educational program states that it is "specially designed to help Orthopedic surgeons in the planning and execution of surgeries," enabling participants to "import digital images, size the images, draw out fracture fragments and move them to reduced positions."[259pl] The online app places "implants sized precisely to your x-rays or digital Pacs systems images from the comfort of your IPAD, tablet, computer or phone," and produces processes, as well as sizes and types of surgical tools needed, potentially reducing waste.[263] The Bonesetter App can also aid in the training of residents by allowing them to plan and review step-by-step measures needed (prior to) conducting these orthopedic surgeries.

In a follow-up 2022 study, the Bonesetter App was used by orthopedic practitioners to measure alignment and malalignment of lower limb axial deformities using the online digital tool. The study showed

56%—84% success rate range among the four case studies provided to the participating orthopedic surgeons.[263] Clearly, such innovative approaches to surgical orthopedic instruction can help LMICs bridge their 'geographical gap' by learning new skills, identifying errors in measurements, differentiating between anteversion (rotates inward) and retroversion (rotates outward) of the femur, and reducing expensive in-person training and travel costs.

25. Implement **Patient-Centered Care Charter** and objectives for hospitals and clinics. Understandably, the low patient-to-provider ratios in Africa constrain available time(s) spent with patients. However, there can be a palpable lack of patient-centered care (PCC) displayed in many sub-Saharan hospital wards and physician's offices. General finger-pointing for these chronic gaps can be aimed at one, some, or all of the following: staff shortages, policy inertia, outdated/Colonial-era patient care models, low staff motivation, inadequate supervision, inadequate staff training in communication, limited accountability in the provision of care, and poor infrastructure to ensure patient confidentiality and protection of privacy.[241] Additional issues can also include the elimination of hierarchical and/or patriarchal cultural norms (only the aged male 'doctor knows best'); increased patient involvement (self-efficacy), poor staff training in communication, limited accountability in the provision of care, and poor infrastructure to ensure patient confidentiality and protection of privacy.

    The authors strongly encourage the creation of a Patient Charter of rights and responsibilities for hospitals and clinics to widely display, promote, and enforce. The Patient Charter "rights of the patient" could include: 1) the right to equitable access to healthcare (from diagnosis to completion of treatment) regardless of resources, race, gender, age, language, legal status, religious beliefs, sexual orientation, culture or health status; 2) the right to high-quality care with dignity (care devoid of stigma, prejudice or discrimination); 3) the right to truthful information (treatment costs, possible side effects, and risks, alternative options available, diagnosis, prognosis, etc.); 4) the right to your medical records, a second opinion, and/or refusal of intervention(s); and 5) the right to patient safety and confidentiality. Conversely, within the Patient Charter, the patient would also need to uphold several responsibilities: 1) to share truthful information (present health, past illnesses, any allergies, etc.); 2) to comply with all prescribed and agreed-upon treatment regimens (and be sure all protocols are clearly understood); 3) be respectful in your language and your actions to all healthcare providers and all clinic/hospital personnel (no verbal or physical abuse will be tolerated); 4) remain thoughtful and mindful of your fellow patients at all times (who are also ill and recovering); 5) follow all mandated regulations set by the facility, security, staff, and administration (wear a mask, wash your hands, etc.); 6) do not destroy, misuse, handle, steal, or try to operate/manipulate any hospital/clinic equipment, supplies, and property; and 7) should the patient abuse or refuse to abide by any of the following responsibilities, the hospital/clinic has the right to refuse any further (non-life-threatening) care.

In fact, in 2021, the Patient-Centered Care Movement Africa (PaCeM-Afro) was introduced at the WHO's 74th World Health Assembly. On its website *pacemafro.org*, PaCeM-Afro teaches students hoe to embrace patient-centered care, fostering thought leadership in their communities, while advocating for the visibility and implementation of patient-centered care practices among African communities and policymakers.

26. Invest in a national **Post-Fracture Nutritional Supplement Program**. These programs could be financially supported via corporate donors, Physical Therapy companies, NGOs, government feeding programs, etc. While there should, obviously, be an emphasis on what fracture patients should eat (sardines, dairy, and leafy greens—See Chapter 7 "Malnutrition"), it is just as important to educate the public on what foods and drinks and herbal remedies to avoid (that cause your body to lose calcium) like alcohol, caffeine, smoking, dark sodas, and salt. We encourage a dietitian-led interdisciplinary coalition be formed to bridge the knowledge gap among current hospital staff, patients, and healthcare providers, as well as the provision of oral nutritional supplements for patients who can tolerate them.

27. **Fracture prevention** efforts can be targeted at the highest at-risk groups, namely young men and the aged. For the aged, widespread injury–prevention programs can highlight screenings and treatment for osteoporosis (especially for low-trauma fractures among age 60+ females). For the past few decades, high-income countries (like Japan) have noted a huge rise in their aged population, it is now time for LMICs to also undergo the same significant change. According to the WHO's "Ageing and Health" 2024 report, by 2030, 1 in 6 people in the world will be aged 60+, surging from 1 billion (2020) to 1.4 billion; and by 2050, the world's population aged 60+ will double to 2.1 billion.[242] The same WHO report stated that populations 80 years or older is expected to triple between 2020 and 2050, hitting 426 million, with 2/3 of the world's population 60+ years living in low- and middle-income countries.[242]

In the November 19, 2024 article: "Why Senior Weight Lifting Is the Secret to Healthy, Active Aging, According to Physical Therapists:

It's Never Too Late to Build Strength," Tavel explains that women, in particular, start losing muscle after 30, with loss speeding up considerably after menopause (low hormone levels), directly impacting bone health.[244] Exercise classes for women aged 60+ should be offered with slow, controlled resistance and bodyweight exercises that build strength (without unnecessary twisting and strain), such as bodyweight squats, resistance band work, and/or moderate weight lifting.[244] Again, any safe movement(s) for the elderly that are weight-bearing and promote strength, posture, and/or balance (or all at once) can help to stave off conditions like osteopenia and osteoporosis (that can lead to bone fractures), better regulate blood sugar and metabolism, improve balance and coordination (that can decrease frequency, acuity, and/or likelihood of falls).

Conversely, the other very high-risk fracture group is made up of young male drivers (between 18 and 30), who could undergo a specialized 'SAFE' driver training and receive cheaper insurance rates and/or sticker designating them as a 'SAFE' driver on their taxis, *tro-tros, bajaj,* etc. No matter the moniker used, these SAFE driver certification for young drivers must prioritize *both* vehicle maintenance and safe driving practices. Some training modules would include: no previous driving/over-speeding violations; a review of all road rules and regulations; seatbelt safety; driving defensively (lookout for potential hazards and be prepared to take evasive action; 'two car-length' rule (for every 10 mph of speed, keep one car-length between you and the vehicle in front of you); keep a safe following distance from the vehicle in front; don't drink and drive; no mobile phone use + driving, 'Road Rage' anger control, basic vehicle maintenance checkups, etc. Additionally, any misconceptions or myths that people who wear eyeglasses have 'spoiled' vision must be eradicated from the public mindset. At the very minimum, every driver should be tested for a 20/40 visual acuity standard or higher (intermittent checks can be conducted at bus depots and taxi stands). Radio talk shows should educate the public on public transportation drivers who wear prescription eyeglasses are, in fact, a greater guarantee for passenger safety than others who don't bother undergoing annual vision screening.

Plus, every time a driver of a public vehicle gets ready to pick up passengers, they should check the roadworthiness of their vehicle by checking that: windscreen, windows, and mirrors are undamaged and clear; seatbelts are available; all headlights, brake lights, signals, horn, and brakes are functioning properly; rotate tires every 5,000–7,000 miles; check fluid levels on oil, transmission, radiator (water), brakes, battery, window wash fluid; check tire pressure; plus conduct a visual exam of tire tread depth (consensus indicates a minimum of 1.6 mm across the mid three-quarters and around the entire tire. Driving 'bald' tires can lead flats, punctures, complete 'blowouts', and deadly accidents. An American life hack is the tire tread penny test, whereby a penny is placed on the shallowest tread (groove) on the tire with Lincoln's head upside down and facing you—if Lincoln's entire head is visible (<2/32 inches), then it is time to purchase new tires.

Back in the 1970s, there was a juvenile crime prevention program called "Scared Straight" in the United States where at-risk teenagers spent an intensive one-day session in a prison. Having seen the unvarnished truth of prison life firsthand, many of the teens were 'scared straight' and reformed their errant lifestyle choices in order to avoid any future prison sentence. By the same token, young teen drivers who continue to drive recklessly, with a wanton disregard for the safety of those around them, should be forced to attend a full day in their local hospital's orthopedic ward, speaking to the drivers who wished they had slowed down, not caused a three-car pileup, fully stopped at the "stop" sign, not killed a pedestrian while driving drunk, and so on.

28. Commit resources to a widely distributed **Public Health awareness campaign** that focuses on early patient presentation for open/closed fracture symptoms (swelling, visible bone, redness, pain), improperly splinted limb symptoms, and the necessary role X-rays play in fracture diagnosis, reduction, and treatment. For instance, in Cameroon, "African Traditional Medicine Day" is August 31, organized by the Ministry of Health, Ministry of Forestry and Wildlife, Ministry of Research and Innovation, Ministry of Higher Education, along with medicinal plant researchers and local traditional healers.[3] The one-day event is used to help strengthen ties between biomedical 'Western' health practitioners and traditional (or tradi-practitioners). Much like any professional conference, there are annual themes (such as "The Role of Traditional Health Practitioners in Primary Healthcare Management"), roundtable discussions, ethical debates, and patient concerns within the practice of traditional medicine.

    Another example is found in Lagos, Nigeria, on St. Joseph's modern Physiotherapy Clinic's public blog, aptly titled: "*Can I See a Traditional Bone Setter*?". The clinic explains in simplified colloquial language that bonesetters hold a cultural place in society, but their services can be risky, and that patients with fractures should go to a hospital instead.[245] Inspired public blogs such as these do so much to help educate and elucidate the all-too-secretive 'why' of bonesetter treatment considerations for the public at large.

Yet another example of a notable research and outreach national campaign is found in Hawassa, Ethiopia. In July 2021, the AO Alliance, along with eight local hospitals, launched a comprehensive campaign for Bonesetter Associated Disability (BOSAD) at the Department of Orthopedics and Traumatology at Hawassa University Comprehensive Specialized Hospital. BOSAD is a "national web-based data collection platform on the practice and complication of traditional bone setting for musculoskeletal injury in Ethiopia"; collecting national data on the practice and complications of TBS, advocating for a "newly trusted modern medical care," and creating a platform for modern musculoskeletal injury care—with their ultimate goal to reduce the "practice and complications of Traditional Bone Setting by 60% by 2030."[246p1] With their motto: "NO MORE DISABILITY ACCEPTED FROM TRADITIONAL BONE SETTING" prominently displayed in all caps on their website, BOSAD (https://bosadstudy.com) shares about 20 case studies from the data collection at eight large area hospitals, including Gondar, Bahirdir, Hiwassa, Assele, Jima, Jigiiga, Wachemo, and Haromiya.[246]

In our final chapter, we will summarize our findings and recommendations, focusing on how the 'big picture' of decreasing poor TBS–patient outcomes while increasing cooperative community-care field foot-soldiers may prove to be the win-win scenario for both the at-risk patient and the healthcare community.

Chapter 10

FACING FORWARD

The 'Human Right to Health' has long been argued as a clash between the 'bottomless pit' of cost objection vs. protections against 'standard threats' to health. As Jonathan Wolff wrote in 2012 in his "The Demands of the Human Right to Health," the human right to health has "been established in international law since 1976" by the United Nations via the International Covenant on Civil and Political and the International Covenant on Economic, Social and Cultural Rights, a legally binding document which effected to "recognize the right of everyone to the enjoyment of the highest attainable standard of physical and mental health."[247p221] As there are many 'determinants of health' (genetic disposition, behavior, physical environment (clean air/water), social/economic factors (income, education, housing), access to care, cultural influences, nutrition, housing, etc.), by definition, the right to health is not explicitly deemed as the right to health care. For instance, some big-ticket orthopedic surgeries, pricey cancer treatments, and brand-new drugs are ruled out of national insurance schemes as they are not 'cost effective'—in that they "do not provide enough health gain," measured in quality-adjusted life years (QALYS), "for the money they will cost."[247p227] Inevitably, these public expense vs. private benefit analyses cost lives and exacerbate the ongoing global discourse on the right to life and right to health, especially in marginalized LMICs. And even though the concept of cost-effectiveness may remain an essential component within the equitable allocation of (limited) health resources, it can be a damning 'test for access' among patients in extremely impoverished countries. The predominance of cost-effective analysis in resource-poor settings can prove fatalistic, and oftentimes, run in direct opposition to the pursuit of the 'highest attainable' standard of health for all. It is a tragic fact that the privatization of hospitals and pharmaceutical manufacturers has steered industry goals toward financial independence and profits, all but precluding the affordable hand/or cost-free dispensation of care and medicines. According to The Institute for Medicine, there are six profound ethical criticisms of for-profit healthcare, including: 1) they serve to "exacerbate the problem of access to health care"[p1]; 2) represent unfair competition against nonprofit institutions; 3) consider healthcare a business and a commodity, not a human right; 4) some incorporate fiscal/pharmaceutical 'sample' incentives and organizational controls that can create obvious conflicts of interest (eroding public trust); 5) contribute to the demise of cross-subsidization in medical education; and 6) disproportionate political power and undue professional dominance threatens passage of equitable (unprofitable) public health policies.[248] Therefore, to overcome poor public impressions and alleviate public angst, concerted efforts must be made in the future to improve the credibility of Western medical nonprofit providers, and shrink the ever-increasing all-for-profit insurance schemes and other public health expenditure mechanisms. Indeed, recent research points to the growth of the for-profit healthcare market share as "not attributable to superior performance on access, quality of care, or efficiency," according to Jeurissen et al.'s (2020) study, but rather to factors such as government regulations (related to accessing public capital funding), reimbursement (for private capital expenditures), cost-containment measures, and payment arrangements.[223p67] Additionally, the researchers claim that governments are well aware of how capital reimbursement plans "steer" the business of health—either toward the commercialization and privatization of care or away from it.[223p67]

Many of the twentieth century's greatest life-saving interventions—from organ transplantation and open-heart surgery to laser and laparoscopic surgery—were surgical techniques and devices, and the technological explosion of the twenty-first century leaked into surgery, leading to procedures never previously thought possible. Perhaps the words of one medical historian are correct: "Surgeons have always been quick to adapt to new technology [...] it should perhaps be noted that physicians were rather [more] tardy."[169p122] As surgery continues to advance, cases that involve minimal access, laparoscopic instruments, and even robotics are becoming ever-more common. Internists have even begun to take up certain surgical techniques. As some examples: Cardiologists can place stents in the coronary arteries and perform femoral cut-downs to gain access to the aorta; gastroenterologists use endoscopes to look at and treat almost all the parts of the digestive tract and to place feeding tubes; and interventional radiologists drain abscesses, insert and remove feeding tubes, break up clots, and even fix aortic aneurysms using various endovascular techniques.[169] Internists and other medical specialists can no longer be said to diagnose and treat illnesses using only their knowledge of physiology and pharmacology.

Drawing Analogies

At this point, it is a thought-provoking construction to draw analogies between the historical physician vs. surgeon rift, Traditional Birth Attendant vs. physician dispute, and the Traditional Bonesetter vs. physician. Like so many other cultural practices, traditional bone setting and traditional birth attendant procedures began as no more than communal spheres of collected successful and unsuccessful treatment experiences, moving step by step into a globally accepted practice of primary (low risk, rudimentary, non-surgical) medical care praxes. Any favorable changes to these praxes are most likely to occur when communities actively participate in constructive education, communication, and social mobilization efforts. Currently, the systemic impact of trained Traditional Birth Attendants (TBAs) to alleviate burgeoning obstetrical patient numbers, hospital/clinic overcrowding, as well as the continuity of wellness care by a midwife for both mother and child—has proven phenomenal. And therein remains the positive expectancies of allowing the integration of TBS into the orthodox fold. Certainly, it bears significant expenditures of time and efforts into working trials should both of these contentious segments embrace the (rather inevitable) alterations to their social roles and professional reputations.

Unfortunately, most medical and scientific changes occur not because individual scientists or physicians are successful in shifting some putative viewpoint, but rather through the successive generations of physicians and scientists who gradually are able to bring a divergent viewpoint. To paraphrase German physicist Max Planck: Science advances one funeral at a time. Or more precisely, Planck stated: "A new scientific truth does not triumph by convincing its opponents and making them see the light, but rather because its opponents eventually die, and a new generation grows up that is familiar with it."[250p33] Planck also added that: "An important scientific innovation rarely makes its way by gradually winning over and converting its opponents: it rarely happens that Saul becomes Paul," and that what happens is that "its opponents gradually die out, and that the growing generation is familiarized with the ideas from the beginning: another instance of the fact that the future lies with the youth."[250p97] So, certainly, as African generations advance—or retreat—from the concepts of fracture treatment options, a contemporary consensus will be achieved based upon each successive generation's reception, acceptance, and implementation of current medical theories.

Conversely, while Western-trained practitioners may recognize the 'chemical importance' of an herb's active ingredients, they may be too quick to dismiss (or underestimate) any holistic spiritual, mental, cultural, and/or societal impact(s) of a traditional healer's care. While it is clear that the TBS practice enjoys widespread community acceptance, patient welfare warning alarms continue to be echoed and reechoed by orthopedic surgeons and Orthodox healthcare community members; lamentably, these clanging alarm bells remain unheeded, censored, and suppressed. Despite this, few traditional sub-Saharan African healers or bonesetters are officially recognized, resgistered, certified, or standardized by national medical boards, NGOS, and/or government organizations, operating well outside any legal or ethical parameters of formal health systems—without concerns of civil or criminal penalties, accountability, or responsibilities. Therefore, these consequence-free healers remain blissfully immune, and unencumbered by laws, ethics, or social justice imperatives. As a global healthcare community, we must ask ourselves if traditional bonesetters who too tightly splint, carelessly administer contaminated and/or toxic substances, advertise misleading 'miracle cures' and 'instant healings' be allowed to continue to cripple, maim, or permanently disable innocent pediatric patients and adults? Of course not. But it behooves each nation's Ministry of Health to reflect on the core tenets, *the very marrow if you will*, of bone healing—and how the treatment offered by some traditional bonesetters violates these evidence-based scientific principles. But the positive exploitation of the TBS's natural herbal resourcing and regional patient familiarities may in many ways prove informative—perhaps even edifying—to us as modern-day practitioners. Perhaps if given appropriate skills and means, they can be well placed to take on even larger roles in combating Africa's ever-growing Burden of Injuries.

As for economics, there is iron-clad documented evidence showing that it is reckless and fiscally irrational for any nation to forfeit its principal custodian of power, success, and wealth—its citizens—to disability, malnutrition, sickness, and substandard health education. To be fair, of course Western orthodox physicians are not infallible and make errors in diagnosis and treatment. The indisputable difference is that nationally recognized healthcare providers are held accountable, both civilly and criminally, for any malicious harm, gross negligence, repeat offenses, fraudulent billing, or irresponsible actions. For these offenses, providers are publicly discredited via a loss of their medical license by their professional peers, their freedom (jail), and their livelihood (ability to work as a physician).

To reiterate, the overriding purpose for this work has never changed for us—as physicians, surgeons, and researchers—to achieve, wherever and whenever, more efficacious and successful patient outcomes that are timely, responsive, equitable, and safe. At its core, fracture care—much like any treatment option in public health—is never a "zero-sum" scheme. So, it's important to remember that the gains of one party are not exactly balanced by the losses of the other, with no 'net benefit' created. Therefore, a more responsive and reactive community mindset and Public Health educational curriculum could, conceivably, bolster patient-centric care—empowering communities to purge themselves of unregulated cons that openly (and with the public's tacit consent) rip off citizens of their hard-earned salaries and rob them of a lifetime of good health. Again, we are not condoning 'throwing the baby out with the bathwater', but rather reforming and integrating traditional bonesetters' treatment regimens to "first do no harm," work as regulated community-level providers, safely uplifting the public's wellbeing.

To conclude, there's an accepted time-worn adage begun by Densen in 2011, that hypothesizes the "amount of medical knowledge is said to double every 73 days."[251p50] Therefore, considering medicine's mercurial, ever-changing environ, surely there must be some designated spaces for measured African regional, national, and even global, fracture-care considerations and transformations toward more efficacious and successful patient outcomes that are timely, responsive, equitable, and safe.

REFERENCES

1. Bishaw M. Promoting traditional medicine in Ethiopia: a brief historical review of government policy. *Soc Sci & Med.* 1991;33(2):193–200.
2. Libretti S, Puckett Y. *Physiology, Homeostasis.* StatPearls [Internet]. StatPearls Publishing; 2024. www.ncbi.nlm.nih.gov/books/NBK559138
3. Fokunang CN, Ndikum V, Tabi OY, Jiofack RB, Ngameni B, Guedje NM, Tembe-Fokunang EA, Tomkins P, Barkwan S, Kechia F, Asongalem E, Ngoupayou J, Torimiro NJ, Gonsu KH, Sielinou V, Ngadjui BT, Angwafor F, Nkongmeneck A, Abena OM, Ngogang J, Asonganyi T, Colizzi V, Lohoue J, Kamsu-Kom. Traditional medicine: past, present and future research and development prospects and integration in the National Health System of Cameroon. *Afr J Tradit Complement Altern Med.* 2011;8(3):284–295.
4. Hillenbrand E. Improving traditional-conventional medicine collaboration: perspectives from Cameroonian traditional practitioners. *Nord J Afr Stud.* 2006;15(1).
5. Fanon F. *The Wretched of the Earth.* Grove Press; 1961.
6. Farmer P. Challenging orthodoxies: the road ahead for health and human rights. *Health Hum Rights.* 2008;10(1):5–19.
7. Hoff W. Traditional health practitioners as primary health care workers. *Trop Doct.* 1997;27(1):52–55. doi: 10.1177/00494755970270S116
8. Onuminya JE. Performance of a trained traditional bonesetter in primary fracture care. *Suid-Afrikaanse tydskrif vir geneeskunde.* 2006;96(4):320–322.
9. AO Alliance. Catalyzing health systems change: training traditional bonesetters in Ghana. November 2, 2022. www.aofoundation.org/spine/education/faculty/facultyfocus-ao-spine/ff-2022-02
10. Nwafor JA, Edet R, Nwokocha E. Beyond borders: exploring the lived experiences of international migrant women in Nigeria, a deep dive into healthcare realities and utilization. *Gend Issues.* 2025;42(2):12.
11. Magesa L. *What Is Not Sacred? African Spirituality.* Orbis Books; 2013.
12. Magesa L. *African Religion: The Moral Traditions of the Abundant Life.* Orbis Books; 1997.
13. Pew Research Center. Orthodox Christianity in the 21st Century: orthodox Christians are highly religious in Ethiopia, much less so in former Soviet Union. November 8, 2017. https://www.pewresearch.org/religion/2017/11/08/orthodox-christians-are-highly-religious-in-ethiopia-much-less-so-in-former-soviet-union
14. Alegbeleye B. Traditional bonesetting practices in the northwest region of Cameroon. *East Cent Afr J Surg.* 2019;24(1):47–60.
15. Forbes JG. The Tropical Diseases most prevalent among the inhabitants of the Gold Coast Colony. *J Royal Afr Society.* 1904;3(12):361–380.
16. Tosam MJ. Healthcare and spirituality: a traditional African perspective. *Annali di Studi Religiosi.* 2021; 22: 255–277.

17. Koenig HG, King DE, Carson VB. *Handbook of Religion and Health.* 2nd ed. Oxford University Press; 2012.
18. Janzen, JM. *Ngoma: Discourses of Healing in Central and Southern Africa.* University of California Press; 1992.
19. Dube L, Shoko T, Hayes S. *African Initiatives in Healing Ministry.* UNISA Press; 2011.
20. Richter R. *Medical Outcasts: Gendered and Institutionalized Xenophobia in Undocumented Forced Migrants' Emergency Healthcare.* Lexington Books; 2015.
21. Gray J. *Ashe, Traditional Religion and Healing in Sub-Saharan Africa and the Diaspora: A Classified International Bibliography.* Greenwood Pub Group; 1989.
22. Janzen JM. *The Quest for Therapy in Lower Zaire.* University of California Press; 1978.
23. Gelfand M. *The Traditional Medical Practitioner in Zimbabwe: His Principles of Practice and Pharmacopoeia.* Mambo Press; 1985.
24. Nkongmeneck BA, Mapongmetsem PM, Pinta YV, Nkuinkeu R, Tsabang N, Fongnzossie E, Kemeuze V, Jiofack T, Johnson M, Asaha S, Sakwe C, Mboufack C. Etat des lieux des plantes médicinales importantes à conserver et des jardins de plantes médicinales à promouvoir. *Rapport CEN/OMS/MEM.* 2007;24.
25. Ecklund EH, Scheitle CP. *Religion vs. Science: What Religious People Really Think.* Oxford University Press; 2018.
26. Kobayashi D, Kuga H, Shimbo T. Slight religiosity associated with a lower incidence of any fracture among healthy people in a multireligious country. *Biopsychosoc Med.* 2023;17(1):3. doi: 10.1186/s13030-023-00265-6
27. Cochrane JR, Gunderson G, Cutts T. *Handbook on Religion and Health: Pathways for a Turbulent Future.* Edward Elgar Publishing; 2024.
28. Richter R, Flowers T, Bongmba EK. *Witchcraft as a Social Diagnosis: Traditional Ghanaian Beliefs and Global Health.* Lexington Books; 2017.
29. CNN. Brain drain or brain gain? Meet 7 African medical heroes who came home to defy death. March 5, 2015. https://www.cnn.com/2015/03/05/africa/gallery/african-medical-heroes/index.html
30. Wane N. The Kenyan herbalist ruptures the status quo in health and healing. *Counterpoints.* 2011;379:280–298.
31. World Health Organization. Road traffic injuries. June 20, 2022. https://www.who.int/news-room/fact-sheets/detail/road-traffic-injuries
32. World Health Organization. Injuries and violence. June 19, 2024. https://www.who.int/news-room/fact-sheets/detail/injuries-and-violence
33. World Health Organization. *From Burden to "best buys": Reducing the Economic Impact of Non-Communicable Diseases in LMICs.* WHO; 2011.
34. Rossiter ND. Trauma—the forgotten pandemic? *Int Ortho.* 2022;46:3–11.
35. Economist Intelligence Unit. At breaking point: understanding the impact of musculoskeletal injuries in low- and middle-income countries. AO Alliance, U.K; 2018.
36. World Health Organization. *Annual Deaths from the WHO Global Health Observatory.* WHO; 2019. www.who.int/data/gho
37. Global Burden of Disease 2019 Fracture Collaborators. Global, regional, and national burden of bone fractures in 204 countries and territories, 1990–2019: a systematic analysis from the Global Burden of Disease study 2019. *Lancet Healthy Longev.* 2021;2(9):e580–e592.
38. O'Hara NN, Mugarura R, Potter J, Stephens T, Rehavi MM, Francois P, Blachut PA, O'Brien PJ, Mezei A, Beyeza T, Slobogean GP. The socioeconomic implications of isolated tibial and femoral fractures from road traffic injuries in Uganda. *J Bone Joint Surg Am.* 2008;100(7):e43.

39. Singaram S, Naidoo M. The psychological impact of long bone fractures in KwaZulu-Natal, South Africa: a cross-sectional study. *J Public Health Afr.* 2020;11(2):1128.
40. Ghana News Agency. Road accidents: a contributor to disability. December 20, 2023. https://gna.org.gh/2023/12/road-accidents-a-contributor-to-disability
41. Sofowora A. Research on medicinal plants and traditional medicine in Africa. *J Alt Compl Med.* 1996;2:365–372. https://doi.org/10.1089/acm.1996.2.365
42. Richter R, Oduro G, Bonney J, Forson P, Oppong C, Flowers T, Richter RW. Utilizing AEMS (Assess-EOP-Map-Simulate) algorithm to assess and spatially link prehospital emergency medical services resources in road-traffic mass casualty incidents in Kumasi, Ghana. *Prehospital Disaster Med.* 2023;38(S1):s130. doi:10.1017/s1049023x23003436
43. UNICEF. Harmful cultural practices. August 2024. https://www.unicef.org/protection
44. World Health Organization. Female genital mutilation. February 5, 2024. https://www.who.int/news-room/fact-sheets/detail/female-genital-mutilation
45. Ontiveros E. What is FGM, where does it happen and why? *BBC World Service.* February 6, 2019.
46. Williams-Breault BD. Eradicating female genital mutilation/cutting: human rights-based approaches of legislation, education, and community empowerment. *Health Hum Rights.* 2018;20(2):223–233.
47. Leonti, M. Are we romanticizing traditional knowledge? A plea for more experimental studies in ethnobiology. *J Ethnobio Ethnomed.* 2024;20:56. https://doi.org/10.1186/s13002-024-00697-6
48. Ewuoso C, Fayemi AK, Aramesh K. Ubuntu ethics and moral problems in traditional bone-healing. *J Global Health Rep.* 2021;5:e2021032.
49. New York Times. Suing a natural bone-setter; a Connecticut Dr. Sweet and the family he sprang from. December 17, 1883.
50. Hong Kong Government. *Definition of Health Expenditure.* Food and Health Bureau of the Government of the Hong Kong Special Administrative Region; 2018.
51. Epker E. Truly unsustainable: the effect of medical malpractice on caregiving. *Forbes.* July 18, 2024.
52. Hippocrates. *The Oath. Hippocratic Oath.* William HS Jones, trans. 1923:147.
53. Hippocrates. *The Hippocratic Oath.* Lasagna L, trans. Dalhousie University Library; 1964. https://dal.ca.libguides.com/c.php?g=256990&p=1717826
54. Azmand S, Heydari M. Medical ethics according to Avicenna's stance: a synopsis. Galen Med J. 2018;6.
55. Yasin SM, Ayana B, Bezabih B, Wamisho BL. Causes of pediatric limb amputations at Tikur Anbessa Hospital and the role of traditional bone setters "Wogeshas". *Ethiop Med J.* 2018;56(2).
56. Idris S, Mohammed O, Basheer E. Why do people prefer traditional bonesetters in Sudan? *Sudan J Med Sci.* 2010;5(3).
57. Nwachukwu BU, Okwesili IC, Harris MB, Katz JN. Traditional bonesetters and contemporary orthopedic fracture care in a developing nation: historical aspects, contemporary status and future directions. *Open Orthop J.* 2011;7(5):20–26. doi:10.2174/1874325001105010020
58. Makoge V, Maat H, Vaandrager L, Koelen M. Health-seeking behavior towards Poverty-Related Disease: a qualitative study of people living in camps and on campuses in Cameroon. *PLoS Negl Trop Dis.* 2017;11(1):e0005218.
59. Dickson DC, Christie SA, Mefire AC, Oben E, Embolo FN, Fonje AN, O'Sullivan O, Akumbu PW, Essi MJ, Dicker R, Juillard C. A qualitative study

of transitions between health care settings after injury in Cameroon. *J Surg Res.* 2019;244:528–539.

60. Akakpo SB. Why patients patronize the services of traditional bone setters: a phenomenological analysis of lived experiences of patients in Ghana. *Afr Social Sci Hum J.* 2024;5(4):2709–1309.
61. Card EB, Obayemi JE, Shirima O, Lazaro M, Massawe H, Stanifer JW, Premkumar A, Sheth NP. Practices and perspectives of traditional bone setters in northern Tanzania. *Ann Glob Health.* 2020;86(1):61.
62. Yempabe T, Edusei A, Donkor P, Buunaaim A, Mock C. Traditional bonesetters in Ghana: opportunities for engagement with the formal health sector. *Pan Afr Med J.* 2020;37:248.
63. Mengistu G, Gebrehana E, Gari T, Bussa S, Alemu E, Zerihun Y, Wude Z, Harrison W. Being children and delayed presentation are main risk factors for developing complications following traditional bone setting in southern Ethiopia. *Eth Med J.* 2024;62:47–53.
64. World Bank Group. Current health expenditure (% of GDP) World Health Organization global health expenditure database. April 04, 2025. apps.who.int/nha/database
65. Stekelenburg J, Jager BE, Kolk PR, Westen EH, van der Kwaak A, Wolffers IN. Health care seeking behaviour and utilisation of traditional healers in Kalabo, Zambia. *Health Policy.* 2005;71(1):67–81. doi: 10.1016/j.healthpol.2004.05.008
66. Clark A. *The Impact of Deforestation on Medicinal Plant Species in Africa.* Wilson Center; 2023. https://www.wilsoncenter.org/blog-post/deforestation-medicinal-plant-species-in-africa
67. Fonkoue L, Muluem KO, Nana T, Kong D, Ngongang O, Yamben MA, Tambekou U, Tagakou J. Outcome of a 2-stage management of open tibia fracture in a low-income country lacking plastic surgeons: a retrospective study. *Orthoplastic Sur.* 2023;13:25–30.
68. Onyemaechi NO, Itanyi IU, Ossai PO, Ezeanolue EE. Can traditional bonesetters become trained technicians? Feasibility study among a cohort of Nigerian traditional bonesetters. *BMC: Hum Resour Health.* 2020;18:24.
69. Labhardt ND, Aboa SM, Manga E, Bensing JM, Langewitz W. Bridging the gap: how traditional healers interact with their patients. A comparative study in Cameroon. *Trop Med Int Health.* 2010;15(9):1099–1108. https://doi.org/10.1111/j.1365-3156.2010.02575
70. Ahmad N, Bashir S, Sandhu KA. Utilization of quackery instead of specialized doctors for orthopedic care in district Hafizabad. *Int J Adv Biotech Res.* 2018. 9(1):646–650.
71. Mekonnen EK, Habte BM, Wamisho BL, Yeshak MY. Traditional bone setting practice in Addis Ababa, Ethiopia: perspectives of trad bone setters and ortho surgeons. Eth Med J. 2024;62:55–62.
72. Agarwal A, Agarwal R. The practice and tradition of bone setting. *Abingdon, England.* 2010;23(1):225.
73. Zehir S, Zehir R, Şahin E, Akgül T, Zehir S, Subaşı M. Bonesetter interventions and consequences. *Acta Orthop Traumatol Turc.* 2015;49(4):416–420.
74. Lagercrantz S. The splinting of fractures in Africa. *Paideuma.* 1990;36:115–137.
75. Doumi EBA, Hassan EM. Amputations of the upper limb in El Obeid Hospital, western Sudan: role of traditional bone setters. *Sudan Med J.* 2009;45(2):65–69.

76. Davis K, Schoenbaum SC, Audet AM. A 2020 vision of patient-centered primary care. *J Gen Intern Med.* 2005;20(10):953–957. doi: 10.1111/j.1525-1497.2005.0178.x
77. Colvin M, Gumede L, Grimwade K, Maher D, Wilkinson D. Contribution of traditional healers to a rural tuberculosis control programme in Hlabisa, South Africa. *Int J Tuberculosis Lung Dis.* 2003;7(1):S86–S91.
78. Yongu W, Elachi C, Mue D, Kortor J, Soo C, Ahachi C, Ojo B, Ngbea J. Delayed presentation of bone and soft tissue sarcoma of the extremity in Makurdi: do traditional bone setters play a role? *J Adv Med Med Res.* 2017;22:1–8.
79. Worku N, Tewelde T, Abdissa B. Preference of traditional bone setting and associated factors among trauma patients with fracture at Black Lion Hospital in Addis Ababa, Ethiopia. *BMC Res Notes* 2019.
80. Ekor M. The growing use of herbal medicines: issues relating to adverse reactions and challenges in monitoring safety. *Front Pharmacol.* 2014;10(4):177. doi: 10.3389/fphar.2013.00177
81. Zameer A, Vakil SM, Bhat TA, Dhar SA, Khurshid L, Sofi AH. Treatment by quacks still an issue of concern. *Orthop Muscular Syst.* 2016;5:e120.
82. Alam W, Shah FA, Ahmed A, Ahmend S, Shah A. Traditional bonesetters: frequency of complications with treatment by traditional bonesetter. *Prof Med J.* 2016;23:699–704.
83. Okaiyeto K, Oguntibeju OO. African herbal medicines: adverse effects and cytotoxic potentials with different therapeutic applications. *Int J Environ Res Public Health.* 2021;18(11):5988.
84. Fennell CW, Light ME, Sparg SG, Stafford GI, van Staden J. Assessing African medicinal plants for efficacy and safety. *J Ethnopharmacol.* 2004;95(2–3):113–121.
85. Tsalkitzi E, Kitridis D, Heinz E, Hionidou C, Givissi K, Givissis P. The metal in my body: patients' perception and attitude toward orthopedic implants. *Cureus.* 2024;16(3):e56493.
86. American Nurses Association. *ANA's Principles for Delegation by Registered Nurses to Unlicensed Assistive Personnel.* ANA; 2012.
87. Hanson A, Haddad LM. *Nursing Rights of Medication Administration. StatPearls [Internet].* StatPearls Publishing; 2025.
88. Taylor JLS, Staden J. The effect of age, season and growth conditions on anti-inflammatory activity in Eucomis autumnalis (Mill.) Chitt. plant extracts. *Plant Growth Reg.* 2001;34(C):39–47.
89. Huang CH. Treatment of neglected femoral neck fractures in young adults. *Clin Orthop Relat Res.* 1986;(206):117–126. PMID: 3708964.
90. Onyemaechi NO, Menson WNA, Goodman X, Slinkard S, Onwujekwe OE, Enweani UN, Nwankwo OE, Nwomeh BC, Nwariaku FE, Ezeanolue EE. Complications of traditional bone setting in contemporary fracture care in low- and middle-income countries: a systematic review. *Trop Med and Int Health.* 2021;26(11):1367–1377.
91. Garikapati V, Konadu-Yeboah D, Mengesha MG, Marenah K, Harrison WJ. Systematic review of complications associated with treatment by traditional bone setters for musculoskeletal injury. *Trop Doc.* 2023;53(1):13–19. doi:10.1177/00494755221122543
92. Quinn F. *That Bonesetter Woman.* Simon & Schuster U.K.; 2022.
93. Prasad NK, Reddy BJC, Abhishek L, Katyayini R. Traditional bonesetters a curse to orthopedics. *J Evol Med Dent Sci.* 2015;4:71.
94. Tan A. *The Bonesetter's Daughter.* G.P. Putnam; 2001.
95. Green SA. Orthopedic surgeons: inheritors of tradition. *Clin Ortho.* 1999;363:258–263.

96. Moulton T. *The Compleat Bone-Setter: Wherein the Method of Curing Broken Bones, and Strains, and Dislocated Joynts, Together with Ruptures, Vulgarly called Broken Bellyes, Is Fully Demonstrated. Whereunto Is Added The Perfect Oculist, and The Mirrour of Health, Treating of the Pestilence, and All Other Diseases Incident to Men, Women and Children. Also, the Acute Judgement of Urines.* University of Michigan Library Digital Collections; 1665.
97. Bennett GM. *The Art of the Bonesetter: A Testimony and a Vindication with Notes and Illustrations.* Legare Street Press; 1881.
98. Wharton PH. *On Bone-Setting (So Called), and Its Relation to the Treatment of Joints Crippled by Injury, Rheumatism, Inflammation.* Macmillan; 1871.
99. Legato M. *Eve's Rib: The New Science of Gender-Specific Medicine and How It Could Save Your Life.* Harmony Books; 2002.
100. Panigrahi TK, Mishra DN, Padhy N. Fracture management by traditional bonesetters: a hospital-based observational study. 2017. DOI: 10.18535/jmscr/v5i10.122
101. Udosen AM, Otei OO, Onuba O. The role of traditional bone setters in Africa: experience in Calabar, Nigeria. *Ann Afr Med.* 2006;5(4):170–173.
102. Langley R. *Sex and Gender Differences in Health and Disease.* Carolina Academic Press; 2003.
103. Chu T. Gender differences in pharmacokinetics. University of California, Riverside School of Medicine, Riverside, California. *US Pharm.* 2014;39(9):40–43.
104. Galtung J. Violence, peace, and peace research. *J Peace Res.* 1969;6(3):167–191.
105. United Nations. *World population prospect report 2024.* UN Department of Economic and Social Affairs, Geneva. https://population.un.org/wpp/Download/Standard/Population/
106. Scott J, Marshall G. *A Dictionary of Sociology.* Oxford University Press; 2009.
107. Ezeanya-Esiobu, C. The case of traditional bonesetting and orthopaedic medical curriculum. In: *Indigenous Knowledge and Education in Africa. Frontiers in African Business Research.* Springer; 2019.
108. Hagan GP. Water and spirituality in some African cultures and traditions. *Human Dev Vatican, Dicastero per il Servizio dello Sviluppo Umano Integrale.* 2015;1–20.
109. Blesching U. The bone setters of Africa. *Internet blog.* 2018.
110. Fullas F. "Abish" for a procedural pain control in bone-setting. March 2019. https://wemezekir.blogspot.com/2019/03/abish-for-procedural-pain-control-in.html
111. Abebe D, Ayehu A. Medicinal and enigmatic health practices of northern Ethiopia. *B.S.P.E. Addis Ababa.* 1993:419–431.
112. Ofori DA. Milicia excelsa. In: Louppe D, Oteng-Amoako A, Brink M, eds. *Plant Resources of Tropical Africa/Ressources végétales de l'Afrique tropicale.* 2007.
113. Aremu A, Cheesman L, Finnie JF, Van Staden J. Mondia whitei: a review of its biological activities, conservation strategies and economic potential. *S Afr J Botany* 2011;77(4):960–971.
114. Inegbenebor U, Ebomoyi MI, Onyia KA, Amadi K, Aigbiremolen AE. Effect of alligator pepper (Zingiberaceae aframomum melegueta) on first trimester pregnancy in Sprague Dawley rats. *Niger J Physiol Sci.* 2009;24(2):161–164.
115. Zimbabwe National Traditional Healers Assoc. ZINATHA. 2025. https://zinatha.wordpress.com
116. Abang IE, Anisi C, Asuquo J, Agweye PU, Diderot CT, Ikpeme IA. Open reduction and internal fixation by a traditional bonesetter and quacks—a case report and review of literature. *Int J Health Med Nursing Prac.* 2022:4(1):21–27.

117. Evans W. Traditional plant medicines as a source of new drugs. In: *Trease and Evans' Pharmacognosy*. 16th ed. Elsevier; 2009.
118. Veeresham C. Natural products derived from plants as a source of drugs. *J Adv Pharm Technol Res*. 2012;3(4):200–201. doi: 10.4103/2231-4040.104709
119. Fields D. What is pharmacognosy? *Medical Net*. 2002.
120. Sharifi-Rad J, Rayess YE, Rizk AA, Sadaka C, Zgheib R, Zam W, Sestito S, Rapposelli S, Neffe-Skocińska K, Zielińska D, Salehi B, Setzer WN, Dosoky NS, Taheri Y, El Beyrouthy M, Martorell M, Ostrander EA, Suleria HAR, Cho WC, Maroyi A, Martins N. Turmeric and its major compound curcumin on health: bioactive effects, safety profiles for food, pharmaceutical, biotechnological and medicinal applications. *Front Pharmacol*. 2020;11:01021.
121. Codo Toafode NM, Oppong E, Vissiennon Z, Ahyi V, Vissiennon C, Fester K. Ethnomedicinal information on plants used for the treatment of bone fractures, wounds, and sprains in the northern region of the Republic of Benin. *Evid Based Complement Alternat Med*. 2022;2022:8619330.
122. Newman DJ, Cragg GM. Natural products as sources of new drugs over the nearly four decades from 01/1981 to 09/2019. *J Nat Prod*. 2020;83(3):770–803.
123. Fabricant DS, Farnsworth NR. The value of plants used in traditional medicine for drug discovery. *Environ Health Perspect*. 2001;109(Suppl 1):69–75.
124. Houghton PJ. The role of plants in traditional medicine and current therapy. *J Alt Com Med*. 1:131–143.
125. Mbaveng AT, Kuete V, Ngameni B., Beng VP, Ngadjui BT, Meyer JJ, Lall M. Antimicrobial activities of the methanol extract and compounds from the twigs of Dorstenia mannii. *BMC Complement Altern Med*. 2012;12:83. https://doi.org/10.1186/1472-6882-12-83
126. Ngueguim FT, Khan MP, Donfack JH, Siddiqui JA, Tewari D, Nagar GK, Tiwari SC, Theophile D, Maurya R, Chattopadhyay N. Evaluation of Cameroonian plants towards experimental bone regeneration. *J Ethnopharmacol*. 2012;141(1):331–337. doi: 10.1016/j.jep.2012.02.041
127. Aburi Botanical Gardens. About the garden. Aburi, Eastern region, Ghana. 2025. https://en.wikipedia.org/wiki/Aburi_Botanical_Gardens
128. Sagnia B, Fedeli D, Casetti R, Montesano C, Falcioni G, Colizzi V. Antioxidant and anti-inflammatory activities of extracts from Cassia alata, Eleusine indica, Eremomastax speciosa, Carica papaya and Polyscias fulva medicinal plants collected in Cameroon. *PLoS One*. 2014;9(8):e103999.
129. VıJ T, Prashar Y. A review on medicinal properties of Carica papaya Linn. *Asian Pacific J Trop Dis*. 2015;1–6.
130. Biapa PC, Agbor GA, Oben JE, Ngogang JY. Phytochemical studies and antioxidant properties of four medicinal plants used in Cameroon. *Afr J Trad Com Alt Med*. 2007;4(4) 495–499.
131. Onoja S, Chinemerem E, Ejiofor E, Madubuike G, Maxwell E, Ndukaku OY, Anaga A. Antioxidant, anti-inflammatory and anti-nociceptive properties of hydro-methanol extract of Eremomastax Speciosa leaf. *Afr J Trad Comp Alt Med*. 2017;14:56–63.
132. Valko M, Leibfritz D, Moncol J, Cronin MT, Mazur M. Free radicals and antioxidants in normal physiological functions and disease. *Int J Biochem Cell Biol*. 2017;39:44–84.
133. Finkel T. Oxidant signals and oxidative stress. *Curr Opin Cell Biol*. 2003;15:247–254.

134. Floyd RA. Role of oxygen-free radicals in carcinogenesis and brain ischemia. *FASEB J.* 1990;4:2587–2597.
135. Ethiopia Biodiversity Institute. *Medicinal Plant Diversity.* University of Addis Ababa; 2025. https://ebi.gov.et/biodiversity/diversity-of-species/plant-species-diversity/medicinal-plant-diversity
136. Awodele O, Amagon KI, Agbo J, Prasad MN. Toxicological evaluation of the aqueous stem bark extract of Bridelia ferruginea (Euphorbiaceae) in rodents. *Interdis Toxic.* 2015;8(2):89–98.
137. Bakoma B, Berké B, Eklu-Gadegbeku K, Agbonon A, Aklikokou K, Gbeassor M, Creppy EE, Moore N. Acute and sub-chronic (28days) oral toxicity evaluation of hydroethanolic extract of Bridelia ferruginea Benth root bark in male rodent animals. *Food Chem Toxicol.* 2013;52:176–179.
138. Kimura S, Tung YC, Pan MH, Su NW, Lai YJ, Cheng KC. Black garlic: a critical review of its production, bioactivity, and application. *J Food Drug Anal.* 2017;25(1):62–70.
139. Tran G, Pham T, Trinh N. *Black Garlic and Its Therapeutic Benefits, Medicinal Plants—Use in Prevention and Treatment of Diseases.* IntechOpen; 2019.
140. Aminuddin M, Partadiredja G, Sari D. The effects of black garlic (Allium sativum L.) ethanol extract on the estimated total number of Purkinje cells and motor coordination of male adolescent Wistar rats treated with monosodium glutamate. *Anatom Sci Int.* 2014;90(2):75–81.
141. Amoateng P, Quansah E, Karikari TK, Asase A, Osei-Safo D, Kukuia K, Amponsah IK, Nyarko AK. Medicinal plants used in the treatment of mental and neurological disorders in Ghana. *Evid Comp Altern Med.* 2018:8590381.
142. Kumar GR, Reddy KP. Reduced nociceptive responses in mice with alloxan-induced hyperglycemia after garlic treatment. *Indian J Exp Bio.* 1999;37(7):662–666.
143. Nugraha AS, Damayanti YD, Wangchuk P, Keller P. Anti-infective and anti-cancer properties of the Annona Species: their ethnomedicinal uses. Alkaloid Diversity and Pharmacological Activities. *Molecules.* 2019;24(4419):1–31.
144. Ndjonka D, Agyare C, Lüersen K, Djafsia B, Achukwi D, Nukenine EN, Hensel A, Liebau E. Invitro activity of Cameroonian and Ghanaian medicinal plants on parasitic (Onchocerca ochengi) and free-living nematodes. *J Helminthol.* 2011;85(3):304–312.
145. Nebié R, Yaméogo R, Bélanger A, Sib F. Chemical Composition of Leaf Essential Oil of Annona senegalensis Pers. from Burkina Faso. *J Essent Oil Res.* 2005;17:331–332. 10.1080/10412905.2005.9698922
146. Irvine FR. *Woody Plants of Ghana, with Special Reference to Their Uses.* Oxford University Press; 1961.
147. Hawthorne W, Gyakari N. *Photo Guide for the Forest Trees of Ghana a Tree-Spotter's Field Guide for Identifying the Largest Trees.* Oxford Forestry Institute; 2006.
148. Blench, R. *Dagomba plant names.* United Kingdom, Cambridge; 2016.
149. Singh SP, Kumar S, Mathan SV, Tomar MS, Singh RK, Verma PK, Kumar A, Kumar S, Singh RP, Acharya A. Therapeutic application of Carica papaya leaf extract in the management of human diseases. *Daru.* 2020;28(2):735–744.
150. Bowdich TE. *Mission from Cape Coast Castle to Ashantee (1819).* Frank Cass; 1966.
151. World Health Organization. Yaws. 2024. https://www.who.int/health-topics/yaws#tab=tab_1
152. South African National Biodiversity Institute (SANBI). Biodiversity. Pretoria. sanbi.org

153. Paromik B, Van Staden J. Ansellia africana: a medicinal orchid species with untapped reserves of important biomolecules. A mini review. *S Afr J Botany.* 2016;106:181–185.
154. Hutchings A, Scott AH, Lewis G, Cunningham AB. *Zulu Medicinal Plants: An Inventory.* University of Natal Press; 1996.
155. Chinsamy M, Finnie JF, Van Staden J. Anti-inflammatory, antioxidant, anti-cholinesterase activity and mutagenicity of South African medicinal orchids. *S Afr J Bot.* 2014;19:88–98.
156. International Union for Conservation of Nature. *Biodiversity.* Gland, Switzerland. 2025. https://iucn.org/our-work/biodiversity
157. Leonard CM, Viljoen AM. Warburgia: a comprehensive review of the botany, traditional uses and phytochemistry. *J Ethnopharmacol.* 2015;165:260–285.
158. Maroyi A. The genus Warburgia: a review of its traditional uses and pharmacology. *Pharm Biol.* 2014;52(3):378–391.
159. Bird SR. *Sticks, Stones, Roots, and Bones.* Llewellyn Worldwide; 2021.
160. Oxford University. The role of homogeneity in research: critical appraisal skills program. 2025. https://casp-uk.net/news/homogeneity-in-research
161. Torday JS, Baluška F. Why control an experiment? From empiricism, via consciousness, toward implicate order. *EMBO Rep.* 2019;20(10):e49110.
162. Di Lorenzo C, Ceschi A, Kupferschmidt H, Lüde S, De Souza Nascimento E, Dos Santos A, Colombo F, Frigerio G, Nørby K, Plumb J, Finglas P, Restani P. Adverse effects of plant food supplements and botanical preparations: a systematic review with critical evaluation of causality. *Br J Clin Pharmacol.* 2015;79(4):578–592.
163. Ponseti IV. History of orthopedic surgery. *Iowa Orthop J.* 1991;11:59–64.
164. Ezeanya-Esiobu C. *The Case of Traditional Bonesetting and Orthopedic Medical Curriculum. Frontiers in African Business Research.* Springer Publications; 2019.
165. Howland J. *A History of Orthopedics.* LitFire Publishing; 2018.
166. Majumdar SK. Corpus Hippocraticum "on the sacred disease". *Bull Indian Inst Hist Med Hyderabad.* 1998;28(2):111–118. PMID: 12596739.
167. Swanson LW. Quest for the basic plan of nervous system circuitry. *Brain Res Rev.* 2007;55(2):356–372. doi: 10.1016/j.brainresrev.2006.12.006
168. van Middendorp JJ, Sanchez GM, Burridge AL. The Edwin Smith papyrus: a clinical reappraisal of the oldest known document on spinal injuries. *Eur Spine J.* 2010;19(11):1815–1823.
169. Aggarwal A. History of medicine: the evolving relationship between surgery and medicine. *AMA J Ethics Virtual Mentor.* 2010;12(2):119–123.
170. Ribatti D. William Harvey and the discovery of the circulation of the blood. *J Angiogenes Res.* 2009;1:3. doi: 10.1186/2040-2384-1-3
171. Hollingham R. How agonizing surgery paved the way for anesthetics. *BBC News.* June 24, 2020. https://www.bbc.com/future/article/20200624-how-agonising-surgery-paved-the-way-for-anaesthetics
172. Kadar N, Romero R, Papp Z. Ignaz Semmelweis: the "Savior of Mothers". *Am J Ob & Gyn.* 2018;219(6):519–522.
173. Lepenos T, Sanoudou D, Protogerou A, Laios K, Androutsos G, Karamamou M. Louis Pasteur (1822–1895), Ignaz Semmelweis (1818–1865), Joseph Lister (1827–1912) and the link between their works toward the development of antisepsis: a narrative review. *Cureus.* 2024;16(6):e62543.
174. European Society of Radiology. *The Story of Radiology.* The International Society for the History of Radiology, *Deutsches Röntgen Museum*; 2013.

175. Wood Library Museum of Anesthesiology. *History of Anesthesia*. Wood Library Museum; 2025. https://www.woodlibrarymuseum.org/history-of-anesthesia
176. Barry BO. Orthopedic surgery in Addis Ababa. *Uni Coll Rev.* 1961;1(1):47–56.
177. Sheen JR, Mabrouk A, Garla VV. *Fracture Healing Overview. NIH StatPearls.* StatPearls Publishing; 2025.
178. American College of Surgeons. Advanced trauma life support. 2025. https://www.facs.org/quality-programs/trauma/education/advanced-trauma-life-support/
179. Hertford Osteopaths. *The rule of the artery is supreme.* Kirksville, Missouri; 2024.
180. Meesters DM, Wijnands KA, Brink PR, Poeze M. Malnutrition and fracture healing: are specific deficiencies in amino acids important in nonunion development? *Nutrients.* 2018;10:11.
181. Denworth L. Healing broken legs faster: putting weight on a fracture within weeks can help it mend. *Sci Am.* 2025;332(3):78–79.
182. Lovesley D, Parasuraman R, Ramamurthy A. Combating hospital malnutrition: dietitian-led quality improvement initiative. *Clin Nut ESPEN.* 2019;30:19–25.
183. Abdoola F, Adu-Amoah HG, Addo BK, Anku EK, Hill LT, Hamoonga BM, Katundu K, Msiska D. The critical care nutrition landscape in sub-Saharan Africa: field insights and clinical commentary from resource-limited clinical settings. *Nutrition* 2025;134:112740.
184. Smith T. The fetishism of humanitarian objects and the management of malnutrition in emergencies. *Third World Q.* 2013;34.
185. deGheldere A, Ndjoko R, Docquier PL, Mousny M, Rombouts JJ. Orthopaedic complications associated with sickle-cell disease. *Acta Orthop Belg.* 2006;72(6):741–747. PMID: 17260613.
186. Eridani S. Sickle cell protection from malaria. *Hematol Rep.* 2011;3(3):e24.
187. Eshete M. The prevention of traditional bone setter's gangrene. *J Bone Joint Surg Br.* 2005;87(1):102–103.
188. Luhur J, Dharmawan PG, Wiguna G. Bonesetter's treatment in Sorong, West Papua: a case report. *Int J Surg Case Reports.* 2021;84:106061.
189. Reta A, Bitew Kifilie A, Mengist A. Bacterial infections and their antibiotic resistance pattern in Ethiopia: a systematic review. *Adv Prev Med.* 2019.
190. Chelkeba L, Melaku T, Mega TA. Gram-negative bacteria isolates and their antibiotic-resistance patterns in patients with wound infection in Ethiopia. *Inf Drug Res.* 2021;14:277.
191. Kaiser Permanente. Blood thinners to avoid prior to surgery. March 2025. https://mydoctor.kaiserpermanente.org/ncal/article/blood-thinners-to-avoid-prior-to-surgery-san-rafael-medical-center-ophthalmology-191550
192. Lindner T, Cockbain AJ, El Masry MA, Katonis P, Tsiridis E, Schizas C, Tsiridis E. The effect of anticoagulant pharmacotherapy on fracture healing. *Expert Opin Pharmacother.* 2008;9(7):1169–1187.
193. Hasford F, Mumuni AN, Trauernicht C, Ige TA, Inkoom S, Okeji M, Nathaniel EU, Toutaoui NK, Geraldo M, Amadou K, Uwizeyimana C, Samba ON, Attalla EM, Kebede E, Edou-Mbo G, Okoko EO, Alghazirr ZO, Pokoo-Aikins M, Sosu EK, Boadu M, Msosa OM, Maiga S, Mootoosamy S, El Hamidi S, Eddaoui K, Malema E, Uushona V, Soli IA, Diagne M, Gning F, Kalolo TL, Katumba MF, Kanduza MM, Diteko K, D'Amour KJ, Stoeva M. A review of MRI studies in Africa with special focus on quantitative MRI: historical development, current status and the role of medical physicists. *Physica Medica.* 2022 (103):46–58.

194. Dereje N, Addissie A, Worku A, Gebremariam A, Kantelhardt AJ, Assefa M, Jemal A. Association between waiting time for radiotherapy initiation and disease progression among women with cervical cancer in Addis Ababa, Ethiopia. *Int J Cancer.* 2021;149(6):1284–1289.
195. Harcourt S, Echem R. Patella gigantism following traditional bonesetter treatment. *J Med Tropics.* 2018;20(1):74–77. DOI: 10.4103/jomt.jomt_3_18
196. Physiopedia. Ottawa ankle rules. March 31, 2025. https://www.physio-pedia.com/index.php?title=Ottawa_Ankle_Rules&oldid=367457
197. World Bank Open Data. GDP per capita. Inflation Rates. 2025. worldbank.org/metadataglossary
198. O'Neill A. Countries with the highest inflation rate 2023. *Statista.* July 4, 2024. https://www.statista.com/statistics/268225/countries-with-the-highest-inflation-rate
199. Endeshaw D. Ethiopia's birr drops 30% as central bank floats currency. *Reuters.* July 30, 2024.
200. Warren DM. *The Akan of Ghana.* Pointer Limited; 1986.
201. Ogbole GI, Adeyomoye AO, Badu-Peprah A, Mensah Y, Nzeh DA. Survey of magnetic resonance imaging availability in West Africa. *Pan Afr Med J.* 2018;30:240.
202. 60secondmed. Management of fractures: the four R's. https://www.youtube.com/watch?v=rhuGvufT_JU
203. Ali S, Destaw Z, Misganaw A, Worku A, Negash L, Bekele A. The burden of injuries in Ethiopia from 1990–2017. *InJ Epi.* 2020;7(1):1–11.
204. Ethiosports. Ethiopian Athletic Federation. May 30, 2025. Oregon, USA. https://www.ethiosports.com/news/ethiopian-athletics-federation/
205. Mulat A. *Orthopedic Surgeon Who Aspires to Make Ethiopia a Medical Tourism Hub.* Ethiopian Press Agency; 2019.
206. PlacidWay. Affordable prices for orthopedics treatments in the world. January 2024. https://www.placidway.com/article/2047/Orthopedic-Surgery-Cost-around-the-World
207. FasterCapital. Orthopedic hospital cost: from scalpels to strategies, business insights from orthopedic hospitals. June 22, 2024. https://fastercapital.com/content/Orthopedic-Hospital-Cost--From-Scalpels-to-Strategies--Business-Insights-from-Orthopedic-Hospitals.html
208. MediTek. How much does an orthopedic surgical table cost? 2024. https://www.meditek.ca
209. Raghaven P. Orthopedic implants cost less than a third of the surgery: IMS Health. *The Economic Times.* 2017. economictimes.indiatimes.com/industry/healthcare/biotech/orthopaedic-implants-cost-less-than-a-third-of-the-surgery-ims-health/articleshow/59996417.cms?from=mdrH
210. Hartman S, Bischoff L, Tan J, Triolo J. Unraveling the high costs behind medical device development. *Sterling Medical Devices.* January 26, 2023. sterlingmedicaldevices.com/thought-leadership/unraveling-the-high-costs-behind-medical-device-development
211. Rimsys. Class III medical devices in the USA. July 6, 2022. www.rimsys.io/blog/class-iii-medical-devices-in-the-united-states#
212. Countryeconomy.com. Gross domestic product. https://countryeconomy.com/
213. Knowlton LM, Banguti PB, Chackungal SC, Chanthasiri TD, Chao TE, Dahn BF, Derbew MG, Dhar DH, Esquivel MM, Evans FI, Hendel SJ, LeBrun D, Notrica Ml, Saavedra-Pozo I, Shockley R, Uribe-Leitz T, Vannavong B, McQueen KA, Spain DA, Weiser T. WHO: a geospatial evaluation of timely access to surgical care in seven countries. *Bull World Health Organ.* 2017;95:437–444.

214. Madamombe I. Traditional healers boost primary health care: reaching patients missed by modern medicine. *Africa Renewal.* January 2006.
215. Tsey K. Traditional medicine in contemporary Ghana: a public policy analysis. *Soc Sci Med.* 1997;45(7):1065–1074.
216. Birhan W, Giday M, Teklehaymanot T. The contribution of traditional healers' clinics to public health care system in Addis Ababa, Ethiopia. *J Ethnobiol Ethnomed.* 2011;7:39.
217. Adu-Gyamfi S, Yakubu N. collaborative work between traditional healers and medical doctors in coming up with a cure and treatment plan among the Dagomba of Ghana since 1900. *Afr Anthro.* 2024;22(2):178–214.
218. Soladoye SA, Matthew OI, Lawrence AA. Healthcare delivery among Yoruba bonesetters in southwest Nigeria and the need for collaboration with orthodox orthopedic healthcare services: a mixed-method study in southwestern Nigeria. *Yoruba Stud Rev.* 2021;2(2):1–27. https://doi.org/10.32473/ysr.v2i2.129888
219. Nakuma S. *Perceptions of the Role of the Traditional Medical System in National Development; the Case of Ghana.* St. Mary's University; 1994.
220. Barrett B, Marchand L, Scheder J, Appelbaum D, Plane MB, Blustein J, Maberry R, Capperino C. What complementary and alternative medicine practitioners say about health and health care. *Ann Fam Med.* 2004;2(3):253–259.
221. Shashemene Botanical Gardens. Background. Oromo, Ethiopia. https://ebi.gov.et/sbg
222. Physio.co.uk. What we treat. https://www.physio.co.uk/what-we-treat/index.php
223. Jeurissen PPT, Kruse FM, Busse R, Himmelstein DU, Mossialos E, Woolhandler S. For-profit hospitals have thrived because of generous public reimbursement schemes, not greater efficiency: a multi-country case study. *Int J Health Serv.* 2020;51(1):67–89.
224. Groce NE, Reeve ME. Traditional healers and global surveillance strategies for emerging diseases: closing the gap. *Emerging Inf Dis.* 1996;2(4):351–353. doi:10.3201/eid0204.960412
225. Onuminya JE, Onabowale BO, Obekpa PO, Ihezue CH. Traditional bone setter's gangrene. *Int Ortho.* 1999;23(2):111–112. DOI: 10.1007/s002640050320
226. Konadu-Yeboah D, Yempabe T, Buunaaim B, Dun A, Konadu P, Owusu R, Arthur J, Osei F, Nuertey B, Mensah N.K., Odom S.F., Addo-Larbi W, Martin C, Buehler P, Addo R, Yankyera B, Osei PK, Azaglo H, Martin MS, Okyere P, Mensah B, Misbahu Y, Hamdiyat A, Yeminu B, Mengist B. Clinical outcomes and predictors of patients with fracture in Debre Markos Hospital, Ethiopia. *Adv Ortho.* 2022;2022:3747698.
227. National Records of Scotland. The principles of recordkeeping. Government of Scotland (gov.Scot). 2024. www.nrscotland.gov.uk/record-keeping/records-management
228. Buttolph A, Sapra A. *Gangrene. StatPearls.* Treasure Island, Florida: StatPearls Publishing. January 2024. https://www.ncbi.nlm.nih.gov/books/NBK560552
229. Ekpere JA, Mshana RN. *Medicinal Plants and Herbal Medicine in Africa: Policy issues on Ownership, Access and Conservation.* BDCP Press; 1997.
230. Gbetnkom D. Deforestation in Cameroon: immediate causes and consequences. *Env Dev Econ.* 2005;10(4):557–572.
231. South African Biodiversity Institute (SANBI). National botanical and zoological gardens. https://www.sanbi.org/
232. Enimil A. Na forest we go chop? Accra: Graphic Online. April 2016.
233. Telake BB. Conservation of medicinal plants at Gullele Botanic Garden. https://www.bgci.org

234. Kelatwang S, Abbot PG. *Medicinal Plant Gardens: Promoting Plant Conservation or Rural Economic Development.* Department of Water Affairs and Forestry; 2002.
235. Ndhlala AR, Amoo SO, Stafford GI, Finnie JF, Van Staden J. Antimicrobial, anti-inflammatory and mutagenic investigation of the South African tree aloe (Aloe barberae). *J Ethnopharmacol.* 2009;124(3):404–408. doi: 10.1016/j.jep.2009.05.037
236. Global Data. Q3 2024 update: patent activity in the pharmaceutical industry. October 25, 2024. https://www.pharmaceutical-technology.com/data-insights/patent-activity-pharmaceutical-industry/?cf-view
237. World Bank. Developing countries have a path to creating their own pharmaceutical industries. February 22, 2022. https://blogs.worldbank.org/en/psd/developing-countries-have-path-creating-their-own-pharmaceutical-industries
238. American Physical Therapy Association. Careers in physical therapy. 2025. www.apta.org
239. Rudzki T. Are forums dead for SEO in 2024? *ONELY.* July 12, 2022. https://www.onely.com
240. Bonesetter Solutions. Bonesetter app. LLC Ann Arbor Michigan, USA. 2025. https://detroitbonesetter.com
241. Muganzi DJ, Namara CM, Kintu TM, Atulinda L, Kihumuro RB, Ahaisibwe B, Montori VM. Paving the path to patient-centered healthcare in Africa: insights from a student-led initiative. *Ann Glob Health.* 2024;90(1):27. doi: 10.5334/aogh.4250
242. World Health Organization. Ageing and health. October 1, 2024. https://www.who.int/news-room/fact-sheets/detail/ageing-and-health
243. Reynolds T, Sawe H, Rubiano A, Shin S, Wallis L, et al. Strengthening health systems to provide emergency care. In Jamison DT, Gelband H, Horton S, Jha P, Laxminarayan R, Mock CN, Nugent R, eds. *Disease Control Priorities.* 3rd ed. World Bank; 2017.
244. Tavel R. Why senior weight lifting is the secret to healthy, active aging, according to physical therapists: it's never too late to build strength. *Women's Health.* November 19, 2024.
245. St. Joseph's Physiotherapy Clinic. Can I see a traditional bone setter? May 11, 2024. https://stjosephsphysio.com/physio-blog/f/can-i-see-a-traditional-bone-setter?
246. Bonesetter Associated Disability. *No more disability accepted from traditional bone setting.* Department of Orthopedics and Traumatology at Hawassa U Hospital; 2025. http://bosadstudy.com
247. Wolff J. The human right to health. In: Benatar S, Brock G, eds. *Global Health and Global Health Ethics.* Cambridge University Press; 2011:108–118.
248. Institute of Medicine U.S. Committee on Implications of For-Profit Enterprise in Healthcare. Ethical issues in for-profit health care. In: Gray B, ed. *For-Profit Enterprise in Health Care.* National Academies Press; 1986. https://www.ncbi.nlm.nih.gov/books
249. Darwin Initiative. Projects. NIRAS Group, U.K.; 2025. https://www.darwininitiative.org.uk/project/DARSC171
250. Planck MK. *Scientific Autobiography and Other Papers.* Philosophical Library; 1950.
251. Densen P. Challenges and opportunities facing medical education. *Trans Am Clin Climatol Assoc.* 2011;122:48–58.
252. Adjakpa J, Ahoton L, Kobayé F, Ogougbe O. Ethnobotanical study of Senegal custard apple (Annona senegalensis Pers.) in Benin. *Int J Bio Chem Sci.* 2017;10(5):2123.
253. Bennett D. *Research Sheds New Light on Effects of "Betel Nut" Stimulant Used by Millions Worldwide.* University of Florida College of Medicine; 2022.

254. Fekadu F. *Spice Plants in Ethiopia: Their Culinary and Medicinal Applications.* F. Fullas; 2003.
255. Fekadu F. *Interactions of Ethiopian Herbal Medicines and Spices with Conventional Drugs: A Practical Guide.* A.J. Phillips Publishing Co.; 2006.
256. Chichom-Mefire A, Mbome Njie V, Verla V, Atashili J. A retrospective one-year estimation of the volume and nature of surgical and anesthetic services delivered to the populations of the Fako division of the south-west region of Cameroon. *World J Surg.* 2017;41(3):660–671.
257. Darimani B. "Photographic documentation and description of the arts and activities of the traditional bonesetters" clinic of Gwollu Kumasi, Ghana. 2007. https://www.semanticscholar.org/paper/%60Photographic-documentation-and-description-of-the-Darimani/4f30b0c12611e2e16f0e0a4e412c40ef43c25b29
258. Debas HT, Gosselin R, McCord C, Thind A. Surgery. In: Jamison D, Breman J, Measham A, eds. *Disease Control Priorities in Developing Countries.* 2nd ed. World Bank; 2006.
259. Bernstein M, Bunge T, Rosinski K, Kfuri M, Crist B, Knapp A, Vaidya R. Online instruction to measure axial alignment with the Bonesetter app. *Medicina* 2022;58:1079.
260. Ihle C, Freude T, Bahrs C, Zehendner E, Braunsberger J, Biesalski HK, Lambert C, Stöckle U, Wintermeyer E, Grünwald J, Grünwald L, Ochs G, Flesch I, Nüssler A. Malnutrition—an underestimated factor in the inpatient treatment of traumatology and orthopedic patients: a prospective evaluation of 1055 patients. *Injury.* 2017;48(3):628–636.
261. Open Secrets. U.S. Senate Office of Public Records. Sector profile: health. Washington, DC. 2025. https://www.opensecrets.org/federal-lobbying/sectors/summary?cycle=2024&id=H
262. Gullelle Botanic Garden. About the Garden. Addis Ababa, Ethiopia. https://tools.bgci.org/garden.php?id=4538
263. Precedence Research. *Orthopedic implants market size, share, and trends 2023 to 2024.* 2023. https://www.precedenceresearch.com/orthopedic-implant-market
264. Weeks C. Home blenderized tube feeding: a practical guide for clinical practice. *Clin Transl Gastroenterol.* 2019;10(2):e00001.
265. Omololu AB, Ogunlade SO, Gopaldasani VK. The practice of traditional bone setting: training algorithm. *Clin Orthop Relat Res.* 2008;466(10):2392–2398. doi: 10.1007/s11999-008-0371-8
266. Yang J. Annual lobbying expenditure on health sector in the United States in 2024, by sector. *Statista.com.* November 24, 2025.
267. Bhattacharyya P, Van Staden J. Ansellia africana (Leopard orchid): a medicinal orchid species with untapped reserves of important biomolecules—a mini review. *S Afr J Botany.* 2016;106:181–185.
268. Schoffeleers M. *Guardians of the Land: Essays on Central African Territorial Cults.* Mambo Press; 1978.
269. Sichting Shirati. *Bonesetter project.* Netherlands. stichtingshirati.nl/?lang=en#home
270. Hillebrand E. Improving traditional conventional medicine collaboration: perspectives from Cameroonian traditional practitioners. *Nordic J Afr Studies.* 2006;15(1):1–15.

INDEX

www.ingramcontent.com/pod-product-compliance
Ingram Content Group UK Ltd.
Pitfield, Milton Keynes, MK11 3LW, UK
UKHW012328180626
472207UK00013B/5